STAND-ALONE

A Message of Hope

Ronald St George Smith

Contents

A Leading Story:

Hello and you are very welcome. I am going to start this book by introducing you to the association which is seen to exist between Dogs and Humans. There is a bond which is seen to exist between the two and reason or meaning does not have to be understood as to why.

First of all I am going to involve you in hearing of an adventure between both a man and his ever faithful, ever loving dog. I was told of this story by a friend of mine called John Elliot and he told me of it because of its innocence, warmth and sincerity.

Dogs live in the present and don't bare a grudge. They operate with always dealing with things as they are; they don't have the ability to worry – or consider things that happened in the past. Neither do they possess the characteristic to appreciate the future, they can only use the present as a media for existence. They see things as they are.

Bearing all of this in mind, let's start our story; I take you to Australia and the movement of goods taken across the country in whatever direction. John Bell was a road-train driver and his order of progress took him on an established route of constantly journeying between Melbourne and Darwin. Consider; both cities standing at the extremes of the country – top and bottom with a distance of about 4000 kilometres separating them. He would move between these two cities on a continual basis and was a known and established road-train driver.

His rig usually consisted of what is called a B-triple. This is a rig pulling three trailers and is a recognisable feature on outback roads.

He travelled alone and in order to relieve the monotony he would travel with a recognisable companion; his companion of many years, an Alsatian called Mac.

Mac was an endearing 7 year old Alsatian dog who seemed to understand and tolerate the ever recurring moments of solitude which would exist as the Road-Train moved from the north to the south of the vast antipodes existing between Darwin and Melbourne. He had come into John's possession as a very young puppy and it could be understood that after all the years of attachment Mac knew of no other tolerable co-existence then of a life spent with John.

As our story begins, John is intent on taking the Road-Train out of Darwin and heading towards the very far distant city of Melbourne. Mac is contentedly reclining in the small space existing directly behind the driver's seat and considering the coming days of solitude. John brings the vehicle along the Stuart Highway as far as Three Ways; where he will alter his course to head deep into Queensland in order to secure as direct a route as possible for his destination.

Since Darwin, the monopolistic conversation occurring in the cab of the Road-Train had not risen much above a deliberate silence. John was intent upon his driving and Mac had assumed an indifferent posture whereby no space existed for anyone else. They had not yet hit the upcoming miles of tortuous silence with the ever present horizon holding similar lines of extenuating scenery. As was usual when they came to a small township along the Barkly Highway called Camooweal, John slowed the cab along with the following convoy of participating trailers and brought all to a halt at a convenient *watering hole*. He went into the diner for a final meal and left Mac to sniff around the outside vegetation (or scrub) and to perform bodily functions which dogs sometimes have a need for. He concluded his meal and came outside to find the dog. No dog. He searched for the best part of an hour, no sign and then appreciating his self-imposing timetable (Melbourne was waiting) he knew that with time pressing he was going to have to leave his inveterate companion.

It wasn't something which he was making available to himself, he knew that he had searched for the dog and he knew that he was going to appreciate a loss but commerce was commerce. Faceless bureaucrats deep down in Melbourne would be singularly indifferent to a plea from him as to having lost his dog. So with reluctance he boarded the Road-Train and headed south.

He faced the usual silence and lost himself amongst the usual chart-topping singles which had always accompanied him in the past. He faced the silence which not having his 'shadow' was having on him. Very quickly he recognised the singularity which Mac's absence was binging about, but life was life and with his Australian mentality he brought into being a list of priorities. Sorry to say but Mac was way down on the list.

In enforced silence he got to Melbourne, having paused at numerous watering holes. He found that as he descended from the cab mates were gathering around him and expressing an interest in where Mac had got himself to. Hearing that he had disappeared somewhere close to Camooweal, they all assured him that if they were in the vicinity they would keep an eye out.

Months went passed with numerous trips between Melbourne and Darwin. Each time Camooweal was achieved John would find himself looking with particular interest behind sheds and homesteads which he was passing. He missed Mac and would not think of replacing his friend. Far from becoming indifferent he was finding instead that he would spend the enforced isolation which his job entailed, reminiscing on times shared, times when they had been all to one another. He was missing him.

But as time slipped by indifference became a norm. So perhaps you may appreciate the surprise which John involved himself in when on one of his returns to his home (in Melbourne) he heard scratching occurring at his front door. He opened the door to find a very sheepish and bedraggled Mac looking up at him as if he was just going to climb up into the cab of the Road-Train last seen many months before. John recoiled and with instant love and understanding bent forward to greet his old mate.

An enforced walk for the dog of perhaps 4000 kilometres and remembrance of the route to the house, the coincidence of John being home at the time of his arrival and the complete impossibility of the entire story, makes this a true tale revealing the endearing affinity enduring between dog and master.

I trust that you have enjoyed this tale and from here on I will share with you disclosures concerning a nineteen year old and his bond with his canine companion, thank-you.

1. Introducing Characters

"It's just a question of sleeping on it. Tomorrow things will all appear so different." Was this really the required words which would settle and relieve a mother concerned only for her first born? Six months she had lived with the symptoms only revealing themselves in a form which, if for anything else, had only got progressively worse. Stairs were the latest bugbear, the shear block which would be presenting itself to her son. She was always just imagining the challenge that four metres could present to a child intent on merely allowing himself to go to bed.

The diagnosis had been M.S.; A debilitating and wasting disease which carried no forgiveness, no tolerance, no Grace to carry with it and no understanding or obvious compassion from an unforgiving world.

She; a mother, far from being so aware or concerned only for herself, was now in a situation of having to bear the ignominy for another – her son. Peter had always borne his disability with apparent detachment and with a certain amount of indifference. He would reveal being indifferent to his obvious condition and would regale others with humour or disinterest.

"If things go as we've been told they will, well there'll be no need for shoes." Or, "Footballs will not be required eh?" Sanctimonious or superfluous comments such as these would only create an insurmountable bridge between the outgoing boy whom she had known only months before and this apparent wreck of humanity which was now presenting itself for all to see.

An apparently spontaneous length of time in a person's life; six months, was the time required to reproduce this residue of life; this lovely boy who now was revealing himself to this circus, this intolerant façade, this inglorious debacle masquerading itself as humanity. Wherever Peter would present himself, whether at a hospital for recurring assessments or back at school where he was endeavouring to reveal a degree of normality within his own personal life, judgement would reveal itself.

Judgement was a hard taskmaster. It is an unforgiving rod with which to continually present an intended force for perpetual correction. She cried, alone and often. Taking on her own shoulders, the pain and suffering that the subject of the pain was disregarding. Peter sought a defence to bridge the distance between the person he had come to know as himself and the residue of humanity, which was what was all that was left for him to consider as himself.

Six months ago he had known himself to be a person with a future, life had been tolerable (perhaps even good) and then this weakness had afflicted him. His joints and muscles had started acting up. Suddenly they would behave in such a way as to appear to be in opposition to his very intentions. Walking had by now become a task which (by talking with himself) was effected with some difficulty. He knew where he wanted to go, he could see himself getting there but if the little messengers within his body had a wish at variance to his own then nothing would result except incessant shaking.

He could cry, but for what? Who to tell his tale of woe to? Who would want to know or share in his pain? In conclusion, what had he left? What part of reality could he call his own? The pain was real, the shakes actually existed and the lack of strength was his alone.

There appeared no answer. No solution was presenting itself in order to dilute or dissolve physical hardship. He laughed and with the laughter small amounts of mental strain were lifted. He joked, he regaled his friends, who now saw no reason to continue with their pitying and could only treat him as someone who was bearing the scar of a broken leg or some such condition.

He had, as his defence against this insipid intruder, only his sense of humour and sometimes it proved insufficient (people would either find him immature or conciliatory). Six months before, after a game of soccer, as he was leaving the pitch, he was aware of a feeling of nausea and loss of balance. He had put it down to the effort which he had expended in the earlier game and thought no more about it. However through-out that evening and through the next few days, loss of balance was a condition which was to reveal itself on a continual basis. He told his mum and she placing no importance on what he was saying, past it off as just, probably, another male growing symptom of which she had been unaware.

The dysfunctioning continued and on one occasion, in school, it was even suggested, among the staff, that Peter may have even involved himself in the use of drugs. His standards had dropped and although his attendance within the school buildings could not be questioned, his mental participation concerning school activities was now beginning to be scrutinised. His parents were summoned. They revealed his lethargy back at home and with Peters' confusing explanation as to his complete abhorrence to the use of drugs, a medical check-up was suggested.

Months now involved the pursuance of M.R.I.'s, Scans and Oral (verbal) interaction with various specialists. A guess was made that he might have ingested contaminated fluid and that this would result in the lethargy which he was displaying back at home. But his liver was revealing the existence of no such infusion and as regards a contaminant just passing through his body; time did not show this to be happening. M.S. was diagnosed and considered. It would account for all the symptoms being displayed but produced an immediate division; the medical attendants on the one hand, with the family on the other. Was the condition Medical or Hereditary? How had the condition arisen?

Between soul searching and continual exchanges of endless paperwork, no answer was manifesting itself, but Peters' condition continued to deteriorate. Walking had now become retarded and vision was deteriorating. His speech was a physical attribute which he had always valued and when he found (over a length of time) that his presented speech could tolerate the absence of full stops, he questioned the need to even exchange guttural disclosures to friends. Life was closing down.

At home, his parents seemed divided; his mother adopting a conciliatory position, immediately felt that somehow she must be responsible and spent time with Peter as if he were, all the time, wrapped in cotton wool. His father (Dad) had mulled over various options, but concluded that for the satisfaction of all, his available options consisted of either early retirement (he was fifty four) or somehow he might elect to work from home, in order to assist Peter. His position within his company was as an I.T. specialist, giving him immediate access to numerous internet sources for him to investigate what was occurring to his son.

He was engaged in the study of grading the universe, in a particular package working for his senior company of NASA. By his colleagues' sending him pertinent downloading, on the internet, he felt that he could quite satisfactorily work from home. Having made this decision and regarding the closeness of his family, it would enable him to access information which may very well be at variance with medical ethos. He loved his son and dreamed of a time when either Peter would come to share similar interests/pursuits as his father, or moving on with life could effectively cement his own path in life, revealing   an existence which would only elevate Peter to the fulfilment of new and untried roads; resulting in a conclusion which would be to the benefit of the entire human race. And now Peter had this illness.

The family closed in, secure that togetherness and bonding could only stave off the threatening features of some distant calamity drawing close. The domestic situation was rearranged and Peters' association with the house became that of a single floor. Stairs no longer were presenting themselves as an insurmountable barrier which would require the portage capabilities of Dad, whose six foot four inch frame would resort to the carrying of a six foot one inch shell of a silent conciliatory, compliant package of human residue.

2. Introduction to the idea of a guide dog

Peter held an inventory (within his mind) and conceded that life held not too much. There was only so much that could be lived from the inside of a chair. Then Tim arrived. He was, in point of fact, a frequent visitor to the house and friends with all. Not being a family member he could distance himself from happenings within the domestic scope and would give intelligent and unbiased opinions, whilst offering suggestions which the family may not have considered.

"A dog", was the interjection suddenly proposed by Tim.

"Now hold on, just a minute! A what?" Helen inquired, feeling that Tim had suddenly revealed a new and disgusting way to refer to Peter. "A dog may be an answer to intolerable lengths of time when Peter is on his own. Consider; Home Help is both expensive and impractical. Peter is nearly a completely grown young man, who does, as a person, require time out. He is going to look for a value in life and he may be only capable of securing his own, private niche in life by expressing individualism. He may require his own space and some companion, such as a dog, may be the facet which you require for guidance, safety and companionship, for Peter. "

Helen, whilst relieved that her initial opinion of Tim's words could remain just that; hers, was adamantly opposed to the idea of introducing into her house an additional incumbent. An immediate outcome would be the accumulation of hair everywhere and obvious and, unsought for, surprises, found in dark places, was not a scenario holding much joy – for her (being the one whom may very well have to deal with the same).

"All is capable of an adequate answer. With Peters diminishing eyesight, he would more than most, be perfectly suitable for a guide dog and they're superb. Dogs come in all shapes and sizes. Some shed hair at a rate that allows you to constantly be stuffing a duvet with residual hair, whilst if you tried to adopt the same procedure with other dogs – you'd just get cold. Guide dogs come with a penchant for toilet manners, going regularly and where required. Every objection which you can present, Helen, can be answered with a response which will more than satisfy you."

Over time and with defences; on behalf of dogs, Tim was able to assuage all of Helens objections and upon further reflection and consideration it was deemed to be a worthwhile 'gamble' and a dog became the desired companion for Peter. A companion who would allow Peter to retain what facilities remained within his closing down body; his collapsing frame, for which, he alone was now going to become responsible, if he was going to achieve that individual identity which he might be wishing to claim.

Multiple Sclerosis had been very rapidly diagnosed and without a cure for the condition, appropriate medications were suggested. Peter was feeling literally like a guinea pig and knowing that each suggested treatment was only, at best, a guess. He was looking outside of himself and understanding that mobility was, now, not on his side; depression started to rear its ugly head.

Tim had proposed a dog as being a, perhaps, suitable companion for him. But with no previous history of animal involvement before, how could he expect success to stem from this procedure? But the suggestion was as good as any other, so why not? Where to go? There was absolutely nothing impaired as regards Peters thinking, "Only this damned body". What to do?

3. Keith is introduced and Max makes an appearance

Earlier Peter had been friends with a boy from his school and this same person had once disclosed how having a dog and not much time to spend on exercising it or indeed giving it a satisfactory home – with a suitable form of life (or existence), had decided to give it to the guide dog people. Keith (or his parents) promptly transferred the dog to the local society. They, for their part, transferred the dog to a training establishment and training commenced. Months were expended and Max (the dog) was showing signs of passing out at the top of his section.

He was a very gentle short haired golden Labrador with a suitable accompanying temperament. His only requirement from life was instruction and discipline. His training was telling him that he was going to get all that from becoming a guide dog for the blind. The final part of his training, before his passing out, was a medical. He had had a medical check, upon his arrival, but it had been very cursory and immediate with no extensive investigations conducted. He looked a superb dog and let's be fair, "looks can be deceiving". Accepted onto the course, Keith's parents thought that that would be it, "bye-bye, Max".

Progress reports would periodically make their way back to the house, revealing how Max was always displaying a wish to learn more. In Keith's house no time had been made available for such basic instruction as "Sit", "Come", "Lie Down" or "Go". It was all new and as such Max loved it all and was ever eager to always learn more. Top of the class and then the medical, externally everything checked out perfectly satisfactorily. Coordination, eyes, hearing, reflexes and even skin condition – perfect. Then the internal examination (this hadn't been done before). Temperature having been taken and recorded, the examiner turned to listen to the heart. Securing his stethoscope into both of his ears and pressing the business end onto his patient's chest, he immediately recoiled and expressed surprise. "If this dog is not dead yet and he's not, because I can hear a heartbeat, he will be very shortly". Turning to a colleague, he insisted that a second opinion be forthcoming. His fellow examiner confirmed the initial diagnoses. So, in a matter of seconds Max went from being the star of the show to being 'A Has Been', a reject and as a result the suggestion was made that he be returned to his initial home.

Now that was something which hadn't been expected and so "What to do with Max?" Here was a recently, completely trained guide dog with nowhere to go. But the grape vine has an effect and soon Keith's parents got to hear of Peter and his predicament. Two and two equals four! Max was going to very suddenly have a new home, ideally suited to his demeanour. No more would his life be one of non-direction, but it was going to have purpose and direction.

At home, Max had achieved a certain status. He was now a dog with a very clear mission. No importance had been labelled on him during his 'vacation' at the training institute. He was merely being sent there as a way to remove him from Keith's home. Now however he had brought about a situation whereby he was going to be instrumental in forming a continuing friendship/bond between Keith's' situation and Peter with all his domestic constraints

4. Max goes to Training School

While Max had been away training and reports were being sent to Keith's home, the interest which the reports had engendered had principally been one of dismissal. He had been (or was being) forgotten and these reports were not of any significance. It was something that was now becoming a revelation which was unnecessary. It was a continual reminder that this unwanted dog was still having an impact on the initial abode, which Max had started out from.

He had arrived, one afternoon with Keith, having been discovered by Keith coming back from school one sunny afternoon. Immediately his parents were totally against the idea of a dog assuming an additional position within their domestic plight. "There will be no one to look after him" and "who is going to take responsibility for him, look your father is engaged at work, I have the library taking up all my time and you are at school, with soccer afterwards. It's impractical, NO".

Keith however was reluctant to release possession of the Labrador. He had this affinity with Max, (this was the name which he had chosen – after a local soccer hero). Keith returning home, one day, discovering a very dishevelled, introverted puppy and deciding to see what he had just discovered, thought that it would be clever to test the puppy. As a joke he had dropped his soccer paraphernalia and pointing to the pile, had encouraged the puppy to pick up the pile and follow him. The puppy, immediately adopting the makeup of a more seasoned dog (anxious to reveal a wish to learn more) raced towards the pile of discarded attire. Bowing his head, he rolled the surrounding towel around the remainder of the garments and reaching himself to his full height, he fell in behind Keith heading home. Keith immediately felt an affinity for the dog and in between futile attempts to discover his original home and the appreciation of not, himself, having appropriate time to deal with Max, urged his parents to take control. It was considered to be a bad idea. His father was never at home (except to sleep) and his mother was always away, working in the local library.

Keith, himself, was of the understanding that soccer was going to take priority within his own life and that meant that Max must take second place to everything which was now occurring within his private domestic relationship. So it was something that just came about; Max was relegated to a very much appreciated second place; he lost all significance. He remained untrained, unloved and quite simply, a barely tolerated (or even recognised) air consuming body sitting at the back of the house. An idea!

Coming home, one afternoon, Keith's mother had seen the dishevelled dog, out in the area at the back of the house. She started thinking. The next day, back in the Library, she had looked up for a possible solution to the canine situation. The Guide Dogs presented themselves as a solution. Given to them, Max would finally have a tolerable existence, attaining a purpose which would reveal a use which he had so far been unable to settle into. Investigation concluded, suitable transportation arrangements sorted out and Max was on his way.

Arriving at the suggested intermediate locale, he was suitably cleaned up and discovered to be a dog of remarkable physical presence.

Longing to be friends with everyone but reluctant to trust, Max went through a series of insecurity issues. The little girl who had received him when the transportation van had deposited him at the centre was the first to be welcomed into Max's starting pack. Now that he had realised that Keith etc. had no time for him and he was likely as not, going to end up one very mixed up dog, he resolved to ingratiate himself with someone/anybody else, so here goes. But the little girl just passed him off and put him into the care of a handler who just put him into a pen, where once again he was left all by himself. Nothing changes. But this time there was food and warmth – it was inside. He tried to form a bond with the handler but they changed every day. There did not appear to be any stability in his life.

Two weeks had gone by and a change was the result. A lot of things had occurred in the background which Max was unaware of. He was being talked about. His obvious intelligence and his superb condition were the focus of discussion through-out a series of kennels and although earlier on, Trish, Keith's mother, had enquired as to the possibility of Max being given for training as a guide dog, assessment had to be gone through before continuance could be considered. Throughout the discussions, it was noted that, nothing bad was being said about the dog and if his demeanour should reveal his approving disposition for Seeing Dog Training then things were going to be a cert.

Max and his initial nervousness was forgotten and it was determined that he had now become "just another of the boys". He was the friend of all – if you paid any attention to Max (no matter how small) he became, immediately, your bestist friend. This was an unrequired characteristic for a guide dog, but the assessment station in which he found himself would neither encourage nor discourage this mentality, "let the dog become himself" was the stations' mantra. So with no instruction and with an awareness of increased maturity Max saw the intelligence in selective approval. He conceded that as in any canine pack there was going to be one pack leader. It couldn't be him because he was just waiting for instruction (from the pack leader).

He thought that it should be the handler, who operated with him upon him being released from his kennel in the morning. This man was always teaching him new tricks and he could work with him anyway. He had taught him necessary things, such as how to sit when the command "Sit" was given. Lie down when the instruction was "Lie" and how to roll when the word "Roll" was heard. These were necessary instructions to obey if Max was going to integrate himself within the human world and knowing that this was where his next meal was going to come from – Bring it on!

It was being noted how Max had at this stage suddenly become totally centred on one person, although friendly/appreciative to all – there was no malice in him. It was a noted improvement which was appreciated by the powers that be! Max was almost ready for living, what was going to become for him, his purpose for existence? He was being groomed to make himself available for becoming a guide dog.

Behind the scenes it was being decided that the time for Max to become a useful member of society had arrived. Goodbyes had to be gone through and left to one side. It would now happen that associates, whom Max had come to know, and appreciate, were going to be discarded. This was a fundamental and necessary part within any guide dogs life; they would get a handler/trainer, they would join with a suitable candidate for working with and then, years into the association, they would be retired. Upon the dog having acted as eyes for a candidate for a respected number of years, the dog would be gratefully retired to pass out his final years in the peace and quiet of a relaxing and accommodating animal loving human home. So as a result, it would be essential that the dog had an ability to be able to break his allegiance from any disclosed pack leader and assume another. Not revealing infidelity or a sense of not caring but a mature ability to always to be able to move on.

A dog will always adopt a progression through life which presents itself as the course of least resistance. Accepting its own instinctive canine behaviour (and working with that), it is recognised that feeding is a primary requirement. Man has fulfilled a position for the domestic dog, of being a line of procurement for the same. Litter bins and other domestic rubbish are suitable, alternative targets, if food from human hand should not be available (scavenging). Initially Max had found this to be a satisfactory procedure before Keith had been introduced into his life.

Essentially there are two types of absolute predominance which govern a dog's life; the first (and most powerful) is the need to procreate. Every action performed by a dog, is initially governed by this. The approach between two dogs shows this to be understood.

The second in this prescribed requirement is food (a dog could not continue procreation if it was physically unable to do so). It might be argued with some justification that companionship is another requirement/essential for our canine associates. But if appropriate introductions are completed, a dog can move at any time, between packs and indeed it has been known that a single dog can turn against previous associates – in a physical manner and with serious consequences.

However, as previously noted, an essential associate for this continual need for procreation is the ability to sustain this physical requirement and that requires food. Dogs become domesticated (through interaction with humans) and come to understand that food will always be available (given) in exchange for a tiny piece of subservience. This was brought over and introduced into the dogs' psych (it became a natural part of the dogs' make-up), even fierce guard dogs can be bribed with treats of meat. A form of dog could now be brought into existence where the same dog would exhibit almost supernatural abilities in order to gain access to a fundamental requirement – food!

The guide dog had arrived and with it, a dog who was going to exhibit total subservience whilst at the same time having an ability to think. Not an animal who would reveal the ability to merely say "yes sir, no sir", but an animal who would demonstrate an ability to make life-threatening decisions and see them being carried out to a satisfactory conclusion.

Max had arrived at a point in his life where he was now being introduced to his final handler/trainer before committal to a suitable candidate for use of his acquired skills. A working relationship had to be engendered between both parties before training could commence. So (almost) immediately upon Max's arrival at the training centre, a walk was initiated to bring the association of the pair to one of a working relationship. They were both going to learn from this interaction.

The dog would come to understand the temperament and the psych of the handler whilst the handler would come to know the temperament and personality of the dog. All would be revealed but it would require one parameter - time. Training of a dog, in order to bring him up to an acceptable standard for use as a guide dog, necessitates the dog removing his mentality from one of being entirely guided by canine instinct and instead appreciating the need to revert to total human subservience (with intelligence). Now the dog has to reveal being aware of his surroundings and considering the available consequences.

5. Bill is introduced and training commences

Max met his final handler; Bill. Bill was a giant block of a man, six foot seven with a corresponding mentality. Ever aware of consequences but with an ability to disregard immediate occurrences, he was rather looking for a resulting effect in order to gain results. He had a habit of being able to produce desired results, such as were required but not being able to show how they were attained. The psych of the dog always corresponded to the handling/training which Bill brought to the case. His record was one of efficiency and dedication. Upon meeting, the pair hit it off straight away.

Max was brought into an area where Bill was nonchalantly standing considering the latest concern which was affecting him. Not paying attention to the dog, Bill was idly looking through change in his pocket and very quickly the only individuals within the enclosure were handler and dog. Bill paid no attention and this produced puzzlement in Max's mind. He was unused to being so disregarded and to satisfy himself that the other individual, in the enclosure, was sensitive and responsive, he carefully approached Bill. This was what Bill had wanted. By Max coming towards him, he had instilled within Max, subservience which would not have been the case if Bill had immediately responded to the arrival of Max by a coming forward to greet him. By delaying the meeting and appearing to make it on Bills' terms, he had revealed a temporary hierarchy. Bill was now top dog.

Max came towards him, sniffing. Bill stood his ground and when Max was sniffing the back of his shoe, Bill responded with the command "Sit". Ever willing to appear compliant, Max immediately sat (revealing his desire to follow instructions as given out by the object of his investigation). He was now the follower, taking his lead from the handler. With the dog now sitting, Bill crouched down in front of the dog and reaching under his throat, proceeded to scratch the dog.

Whether or not Max was familiar with this form of approach didn't matter. His space was not being invaded and he could now tolerate association with the party being introduced for interaction. He lifted his head, in order for more scratching to occur. His eyes (the gateway to the soul) were relaxed and inquisitive, he wanted to know more. Bill was encouraging this investigation and the handlers scent was one of calmness, tolerance and total patience.

Bill had not made the mistake of immediately upon meeting the dog, running his hands over the top of the dog's head (between his ears) and forcing an outcome which may have been uncomfortable for the dog; resulting in the dog snapping. Far from it, now a situation had been brought about whereby the person approaching the dog was revealing having respect in his approach and the dog could not feel that his space was being encroached upon. The outcome was happiness all around. So with immediate introductions now complete and Max gaining an insight into the working capabilities of a new handler, let's begin.

Bill reaching behind his back and grasping a lead, attached it to the collar which Max was wearing. He then moved towards the door and without a sound, held the dog back from racing out in front of him. Claiming the door as his own he allowed the dog to follow. Rules were being introduced and laid down. Max had the savvy to understand that he was now totally in servitude to the instructions coming from Bill.

The next procedure was going to come from Bill; a tried and trusted procedure which Bill had used many times in the past and which had allowed Bill to command and lead in his position as the most successful handler in the school. He left the school premises and went to cross the road. At the edge of the kerb he stopped and giving a quick tug to the loosely held lead, commanded the dog to sit. As the dog sat, he was immediately rewarded with a brief fondle on the neck. As Bill stepped off the kerb he said "Forward". Max came to know that in response to the command "Forward", he would be expected to move off.

As time (and days) passed by, small tricks and skills were introduced into Maxs' repertoire. He learnt very quickly that food would not be an expected reward – only a firm hand patting the nape of his neck. Food was his reward at the end of the day. Wanting attention from his handler, all that Max had to do was obey a single instruction. Caressing ensued and Max was aware that, yes, he was both a required and a loved participator in the association between dog and human.

They were a long time getting away from that initial kerb. Max had no idea what was happening but for Bill it was a required starting point. Watching Max and the direction in which his nose was pointing, allowed Bill to know what it was which was holding the dogs attention. He expected Max to give his absolute attention to his handler, full stop. From the word go, Max was riveted to Bill. What was going to be expected of him and anyway this looked as though it was going to be much more fun than an existence of scavenging (before having met with Keith) and humble waiting around in case he had been remembered by the same individual. Now he imagined that he was going to have a purpose. Yeah!

Paying attention with intent, Max understood that whilst he was sitting on the edge of the kerb he might understand that no traffic was crossing by his front along the road. Conceding that Max had had time to assess that no traffic was apparent, Bill, giving the lead a quick tug, commanded "Forward". He waited for Max to move into the road and begin crossing with Bill following. Arriving at the far side of the road, Bill pulled Max in towards his leg and reaching down he rewarded him by stroking the dog with enthusiasm and fondness. Reward extended.

Various instructions and ways of conducting behaviour were introduced from this stage on. The association between Max and Bill grew from this point on and all of Maxs' intellectual requirements were now being fulfilled. He loved the learning process and he gave himself entirely into the care and instruction of his recently discovered and now beloved handler.

"Right" and "Left" were introduced and appreciative turns were then expected. "Stop" and "Avoid" carried their own expected conduct, but Max had to begin using his own mind to lead the expected way and avoid obstacles presenting themselves. After a number of months of consistent walks, Bill came to understand that Max was at a point in his training whereby he was displaying intuition and intelligence. It was time to think of pairing Max to an intended candidate in order to share the next part of the remainder of his life.

This candidate did not have to be entirely sight deficient but if a candidate with diminishing eyesight could be paired with the dog, the pairing could be entirely successful because as the recipients eyesight was diminishing, the alacrity of the dog would lead to a pairing which would hold its own form of appreciative success.

It was at this point in time that Max had failed his medical. He was now surplus to requirements and as such, he could not be expected to remain within the training school; consuming food and filling a much sought after position within the training facility.

Bill made very tentative investigations and came to discover that in the home where Max seemed to have come from originally, there was an individual who appeared to be a contact with an ideal candidate for pairing with a guide dog of Maxs' propensity. Keith was a friend of a school contact who had a debilitating condition called multiple-sclerosis. As the condition had progressed Peter had understood that one of the symptoms he was experiencing was failing eyesight which was proving to be progressive and encroaching upon a satisfactory standard of life. He required eyes. Max was at the stage of revealing having been so trained that he could, now, be successfully paired to a person of Peter's capabilities. It was suggested that Peter present himself at the centre in order to find out if the proposed pairing could be effected successfully.

6. Peter and Max meet

The day of the introduction arrived and Peter arrived at the centre in the company of his mother; Helen. Demonstrating individuality, he insisted on standing alone but his mother, leaning in towards him said, "Peter, dear, if you demonstrate being more active and capable then you are, you only do yourself a disservice". It being an unfamiliar area that Peter was finding himself in, he was tentatively attempting to seek the entrance to the building in front of him and not seeing a door immediately available for progression he was fidgeting in an unusual manner. Taking his mother's suggestion he presented his arm for her assistance. Together they moved off and the door was discovered at the end of a pathway and entrance secured. Walking up to the reception desk, they announced their expected arrival. The girl at the desk, looking at the pair, replied that while they were expected, Bill was being summoned and would be with them shortly. Helen showed Peter to an available seat and then sought to amuse herself by studying the available literature and pamphlets displayed on the surrounding walls. Peter had once more withdrawn into his own private world (it was supposed to be okay there; they knew him there and he was comfortable). Minutes passed and then footsteps were heard coming towards the reception desk. Words were exchanged between the girl at the desk and the owner of the heavy footsteps. The girl rose from her chair and talking towards Helen, informed the recently arrived pair that the owner of the footsteps – Bill, was here in order to take them in hand. He stepped towards them and introduced himself. He led them to a room behind and to one side of the reception desk, allowing them to enter, he closed the door, turning to Peter, he enquired as to the familiarity that he (Peter) had with dogs. Peter revealed that to date he had no affinity with pets of any kind, his being in collage and then the work load which his parents were facing. Bill retorted by stressing that the dog, which was going to come into his area of responsibility, was not to any understanding to be considered to be a pet, but rather the pet was now going to become Peter's eyes – a working associate! He suggested that Peter would never refer to his eyes (being perfect) as his pets and that was the way Max was now to be considered. Max had been chosen as the "seeing eyes" which were now going to form a partnership between Peter and the dog. Telling Peter to remain where he was, for a moment, Bill left the room returning in just a moment (showing that Max had been just outside). Peter was aware of a shape entering the room in company with Bill. Max was presenting himself for Peter's appraisal. Max sat, just inside of the now closed door and Peter, being unsure of his expected procedure, remained standing.

Suddenly Bill seemed to remember that Peter was the one with visual difficulties and stepped forward. Holding Max on a secure lead and grasping Peters arm, he gently brought Peter into Maxs vicinity. Not sensing any tenseness from Peter, he moved Peters hand to under the dogs chin. This was what Max had been waiting for ………… another friend. He didn't appear to grasp that if this introduction was a success, it was going to lead to years of association.

So among this quad of people within the room, there was one fully trained dog, one fully aware handler, one deeply concerned woman and one unknowing, untrained individual who were just shortly going to come into the possession of the first. Oh dear.

If Peter was going to shortly take charge of Max, he was going to have to involve himself in a period of supervised instruction and Bill was ready. He proposed to Peter that without further a-do they should go on a walk around the town and see what interaction there might be between Master and Dog. This terrified Helen who knowing perfectly well that Peter had not left their house for some time now, was going to have to go along with her son meandering around shopping malls etcetera with a dog whom he had only just met, supposedly accepting that the same dog was going to suddenly become Peters eyes and produce some sort of normality within his life. This was her perception, but how wrong can you be?

Bill led the way into another room. Here there were two chairs and in front of them a table. He directed Helen to sit in one of the chairs, whilst guiding Peter to the other. Throughout this time Max had remained completely subservient to all that Bill had appeared to be doing. He followed, with ears down and an inquiring expression on his face, he still wanted to help in whatever way he could, but understood that Bill was the dominant force present in the room so he adopted an ancillary role, content to wait and when required be of assistance.

Bill had returned to sit on the edge of the table, facing the two chairs with Max sitting facing the same table. Bill broke the accompanying silence by looking first to Max and then to Peter. "He doesn't speak English. And indeed has never sat an English exam. Max will respond to sound and to movement but it's unfair to expect him to handle a conversation. He will respond appropriately to words because they hold a particular association (or meaning). It's possible to get him to greet you by saying something like 'bonjour', but that doesn't mean that he can suddenly speak French, it simply means that he has built up a value for a sound with a particular meaning – a sense. Out on the walk we are going to partake in, he will respond to commands such as Right and Left. He has learnt to react when he hears the command Forward or Stop. But what I am going to be looking for is a circumstance where Max reveals a potentially awkward/dangerous situation about to occur to you and he successfully negotiates around or away from it. Upon him achieving that then I will know that we have a successful and required working association between the two of you, but remember – he doesn't speak English, he's never been trained to do that, so it is sound and wrist movement that he will react to"

Considering the value and the weight of the pro-offered words, the group broke in order to partake of a cup of tea. Max lay, in the background, aware that his reward was shortly going to come his way, but it was possible that work would have to be completed first. "We are going out, on a particular route, but Max will be responding to my commands on the first round, okay? You will get a chance to see what it is all about, okay? I will be holding you by the arm and Max by the lead, right"? With this stipulation understood, they prepared to go walkabout.

Inside the hall, just in front of the reception desk, Bill along with Max, stood waiting for Peter to become a part of the unit going out on the prescribed walk. Helen was showing Peter how to fit into this particular arrangement, with the dog leading, Bill next and being followed by Peter, with his hand on Bills shoulder. Helen would become a casual observer off to one side.

They walked along the pathway, away from the reception building and approaching the kerb, Bill did a résumé. Satisfied that Max was taking the lead and that Peter was securely beside him, he noticed that Helen was standing back by the gate. With intense interest and a degree of concern she was watching with concerned awareness. Her focus of life attention was stepping forward into God knows what. Bill (oblivious to her maternal concerns) taking charge, he gave the command "forward", leaving Helen waiting at the gate.

The dog led the way, up to the kerb and at the edge he sat – looking around at the area of his supposed continuance. Bill, saying nothing, stood by the edge looking straight ahead. The dog looked up to the right and then to the left, appreciating no traffic he stepped into the road. Bill followed with Peter intently holding his arm. They crossed the road and Max, after leading the way and getting across, without instruction sat on the walkway awaiting direction to come from Bill.

"Right" was the single command coming from Bill? They turned and continued the walk along the pavement. By now pedestrians were having an effect. Appreciating the existence of the guide dog, they were allowing the progression of the column. Stepping to the right or to the left they stepped back from the continuance of the triad, who continued to make their way along the walkway. Max had his nose pointing directly forward and was focused on taking in and being aware of everything. Bill, completely full of confidence, was paying complete attention to his dog. Peter was shuffling directly beside Bill and attempting to listen intently to available footsteps. His confidence was growing and the speed of the progression allowed him to consider that finally he was facing an answer to his personal lack of vision. Max could be the defence for which he had been searching. If a bond could exist between himself and something as insignificant as a dog, his pursuance of a form of individuality was achievable.

They continued the walk. Down pavements and through shopping malls, the promenade was an accustomed route for Max, but as far as Peter was concerned, the walk was new and exciting. All the time he was withdrawing within himself and considering his possible future. He could think that what he was doing, or engaged in, was similar to himself going into a shop and coming out into the sunshine, having a new pair of eyes, life could be proceeded with and yes, it might even become wonderful. Max was an answer.

After the crossing of numerous roads and circumventing various obstacles, they arrived back at their starting point. Helen, who had been straining to discover sight of her beloved, missed his approach and staring intently in a wrong direction was alerted to his arrival by appreciating a dog sniffing her leg and hearing the command "Stop".

The dog had immediately sat and looking towards Bill was looking for his expected caress. He received it and Bill turning towards the incumbent, trailing along on his left hand side, inquired with a smile as to his appreciation of the value of the initial walk.

"And how long until I can command such control and make Max understand how he should operate with me? I think that this is fantastic."

Bill smiled and turning to Helen asked her what she was thinking. "Words cannot come anywhere close to what it is that I am appreciating has just happened. Peter getting to a stage of control similar to what you have just revealed, will allow his life to be turned around, he will be a new person. What happens now"?

"Well now comes the work", Bill countered in her direction. "I agree that Peter may be a suitable candidate for association with Max. If this is so, the work which Peter will have to do to become a satisfactory handler will have to start straight away". They all walked back down to the reception area and Bill handed the lead into Peter's hand, which he had taken off his shoulder and held for him to receive the entire length of the controlling connection. Peter took hold of the pro-offered lead and working from memory, he held it loosely knowing that Max was going to appreciate that with the transfer of his lead the pack leader/handler was now someone new and with the transfer of instruction now being complete; Peter was to be in charge.

Within the brightly lit reception area Peter may have been considered to be in charge, but how effective this was going to prove would be determined by the following minutes. Bill may have relinquished control of Max but suitable instruction was now required. Everyone, in the hallway was aware that Bill had known how to control/command Max; they were also appreciative of the fact that Peter hadn't a clue.

Bill, turning to Peter, told him that he was to spend the next few minutes in getting to know the dog and allow Max to acquaint himself in turn with Peter.

Were the tables being turned? Visually Max could see Peter but all that Peter could rely upon was his sense of touch. With gratitude he bent forward to stroke the dog, Max interpreted this physical contact as a precursor to the handing over of pack leadership and responded to Peters stroking with calmness and affection. He was ready to be led by someone different, someone else now holding his lead. Bill surveyed all this with satisfaction and told Peter that if he was ready, training could commence. Peter smiled and told Bill that he was anxious to do everything correctly and that if Bill thought it to be the correct thing to do "Let's go training".

Tipping a wink to Helen, Bill turned to open the door in order to allow his charges to exit the building. The dog led, followed immediately by a concerned Peter. He understood that he had never before allowed himself to be guided by a dog and that this was going to be an experience which he would never forget. Once they had all attained the outside Bill leaning towards Peter told him that for the next few minutes his was the only voice to be heard and that Peter must make clear and precise commands.

"Forward", Max started off down the pathway. Bill was standing back and within the precepts of the training school grounds was prepared to allow Peter a free rein. Helen was following her son extremely closely and as they left the apparent protection of the entrance to the building, he could be heard to suggest that she refrain from maternal protection and allow the boy to make his own mistakes. In a compliant manner she appeared to understand and adopted a secondary role.

"Stop" was a slightly more confident command issuing from Peter and was followed by an immediate response from the dog. He stopped and looked up towards his new handler, awaiting a following instruction. The new handler, far from knowing what he was about, turning his head towards the initial handler (if only for support) enquired as to the level of competency being displayed. Enthusiastically Bill responded with delight and assured Peter that his competency skills being displayed were more than adequate and then briefly he gave a reason why this may be.

"Dogs have the visual appreciation to pick up the emotional awareness of a handler (or indeed any person/concern which gets their attention) and it seems that with you having no previous engagement with dogs, you are in no way giving off negative vibes. Entirely being open to gaining an understanding of what it is that a dog is looking for, you have therefore an obvious affinity with Max and I can heartily feel that there may be a connection between yourself and Max".

If Peter had had a desire to hear anything from Bill, this was it. A pairing could now occur between himself and the dog. A relationship could now commence between the two of them and nothing but adventures were going to lie ahead. But as was said earlier, judgement now reared its head and Peter had to declare (to himself – in his own private world) that now work would face both of them and work involved the overall taskmaster of time.

Now let's be entirely fair and appreciative of time, it is an area to move along with. It can't impact onto whatever we are doing; it always goes along side, it is a channel. It can be used or abused but never successfully ignored, it is always there and with wisdom it is not to be berated. Peter was now coming to the opinion that his intended success with Max was going to consist of his availing of what time was available to him and if success was tolerated (and permitted) into the equation then total interaction of the pair would bring about success for both.

Bill continued; - "All life, no matter how big or how small, emanates and gives off vibration. This vibration is an electric field with a particular colour. If this colour can be interpreted successfully and understood, then it permits an interaction between the observer and the subject based on that understanding. Dogs have that understanding and the ability to act, immediately, on their instincts to counter any threat or affinity. This brings intelligence to bear in the appreciating of using dogs to allow sight deficient subjects to avail of the strengths which dogs can exhibit. Dogs don't go through the process of conceding that colour holds a particular meaning and labelling it with an individual expected outcome. Rather the colour displayed resonates with a response/reaction from the subject observing. Now guide dogs, search and rescue dogs, and drugs/customs dogs, or whatever, can be trained to the extent of tempering their instinctive response to work in alignment with desired human results. These points can then become an advantageous bonus towards success in a partnership between sight deficient people and the respective dogs".

Having disclosed all this information and being a handler whom all the time was looking for, at the very least, an appreciated and understandable reason for everything, he was happy with his disclosures concerning a contentious matter. But Bill felt that his giving credence to dogs having the capability to be aware of being able to see 'electrical colours', given off by all living matter, had been defended to the full extent of his expertise. Bill was a happy camper.

Leaning with his back to the available wall, Bill smiling at Peter made the disclosure that Peter and Max were now a pair. So with one afternoon of integration and moments of interaction Peter and Max had made the start to a mutual existence. Training and familiarisation would now have to take effect. Peter had inquired as to the possibly of calling to the training centre the next day, in order to meet up with Max. Laughing, Bill told him that Max was now his and as a result the two of them would be leaving the centre that day, together.

It was at that moment that all of Peter's expectations and desires came together into one huge and unforgettable hiatus, a rift or a gap which he was already filling with unimaginable adventures which the two of them were going to partake of. Then Bill had to spoil it all by telling Peter that he did not know how long Max had to live in this world. He told them of the medical which Max had failed and the suspected prognosis or outcome.

Not completely accepting all the implications of what he was being told, Peter, in a jocular manner, turning to Bill, retorted that their joint conditions revealed the existence of two patients. "We're both going to have our work cut out looking after each other, eh"? Bill was sad knowing that his association with the golden Labrador was so quickly coming to a conclusion, but resilient in knowing that all was not lost for the dog and with a continuing life in the enthusiastic and appreciative company of Peter, all could, in some way be working out for the best.

Whatever discharge papers had to be signed for; in regards to Max and his release from the centre, Helen was making it her business to complete, allowing the boy and the dog to further acquaint with each other. The pairing showed all the signs of being one of success and when it came to the time for Bill to say his last farewell to the now fully trained guide dog, doing it with a heavy heart, he smiled knowing that Max had achieved the existence he deserved. New grounds, new lands, new people and new memories, these were going to now become the future for this most fortunate dog. Rather than putting an imagined strain onto his recent associate, Bill just looked benignly over in Max's direction and turning around he walked back into the building.

This left Max and Peter, at the front of the Centre and with an opportunity to share vibrations. Peter whilst having the power of speech (to some understanding) did not deem it necessary to verbally impress anything on the dog and instead fondly stroked him and mentally impressed his thoughts on the dog, revealing a wish to make their bonding a satisfactory one and indeed one from which they could both benefit.

Helen came out of the centre and apart from being laden down with all paperwork pertaining to Max also had things such as his feeding bowl and a blanket which he had made his own. He seemed to have no idea that he was never going to see the inside of the centre again but instead was going forward to appreciate new adventures and whatever was going to be available.

At this juncture, you the reader, may be asking yourself how Max could possibly have been given into the care and command of Peter? Well it was all very trusting and friendly. Max had been diagnosed as being unsuitable for release as a guide dog; to a prospective failing eye sighted recipient. He was going to be returned to Keith's home (given that the training centre had researched and discovered the initial home before the local society had upgraded him to the training centre). Plans were afoot to return him back to Keith's house when a plaintiff request came from Trish (Keith's mother) that a suitable recipient was available, in the form of Peter. The training centre informed Trish that they would take no responsibility for the outcome – seeing as Max had failed their standard medical. She, anxious to remove the possibility of Max returning to them had proposed Peter as a recipient of the dog and with no acceptance of responsibility given in any direction, Peter was (through Bill) deemed to be a suitable candidate to receive Max and as a result invited to the Centre.

7.   Peter feels sorry for himself

Peter was being brought to wherever it was that he was required to go by his father. 'Dad' was making himself responsible for assisting Peter in small journeys, such as to school. But longer journeys such as to hospitals were imposing on his work schedule, but if it was at all possible he would break with procedure and attend the prescribed location.   Initially and not being aware of any alternative, he was physically carrying Peter in all situations which required Peter to move over an actual distance.   This was proving totally self-defeating for Peter, who at this stage was displaying an intense ability for introversion. He was withdrawing into a world to which no-one else had access. It was a dark place. A place where there was never any criticism, only self-justification. No room for a second person and as a result it could be very quiet.

It was in his own private world/space that he would find it to be very insular and self-contaminating.   With only the thoughts and opinions coming from his own perceived appreciation, he could understand that apart from becoming extremely singular, he could even understand that at times he knew that his opinion was one of being wrong.   But he could not tolerate a second opinion contradicting what he was building up as knowing to be the truth. In the absence of an alternative, he would allow his father to bring him everywhere. His eyes were failing, his speech was becoming impaired and his mobility was shot to pieces.   He sensed himself to be becoming an air consuming body, with obviously nothing else to offer life. Hell, he was dependent entirely on people such as his father, his mother and anyone else who could break through into a situation of being of assistance to him. His availing of this assistance made him (forced him to) concede that he was a body which was withdrawing within itself and displaying being incapable. Hell, he remembered being active, being fit, he remembered when he could do anything and now .... nothing, only total dependence.

His father now, six months after the diagnoses of M.S. for his son, was being forced into a situation of having to completely re-evaluate his life and consider the time which he could expend in the direction, or care for his son. His job was a topic of concern and he was taking unusual lengths of time off in order to act in a nursing/chauffer capacity for his son. His employers were entirely aware of his domestic concerns and perfectly appreciative of the perceived impressions or pressure which Dad felt himself to be under. But work was required and patience was only so long. An answer was now required and it wasn't something as obvious as Peter suddenly resuming his initial standard of health. Looking at the situation, he suddenly came to the appraisal that what he was doing was providing a set of wheels, a pair of eyes and a source of companionship for his son. What could be an answer which would satisfy all the given parameters? He had no experience of his imagined problem so no resolving answer was there to immediately suggest itself.

8. Introduction of a Wheelchair

Now Keith had turned up at the house, to tell Peter the latest score to a soccer match, or something. After leaving Peter (who remained in 'his' room) Keith was leaving the house and passing Peter's dad, he bid him a farewell. In exasperation Dad had said, "Keith, what to do? Peter is requiring complete attention and I am just about coming to the stage where I may not be able to provide what is required. I'm looking for an answer and I don't think that one is going to reveal itself. Peter's eyesight can be dealt with – he's familiar enough with his immediate surroundings for it not to be an issue, but mobility is. He's stuck in his room and intent on going nowhere. He won't allow anyone to move him anywhere and he's just withdrawing into some sort of shell. I think he's close to losing it – cracking up!"

"A wheelchair"

Peter's Dad responded with "A what?"

Keith countered with repeating himself, "A wheelchair, it may be the solution to your problem. I don't want Peter knowing that the suggestion came from me but you might agree that it is a solution". Keith left with this thought planted in Dads mind. Dad considered.

Keith had gone home, concerned over the welfare of his, up till not so long ago, soccer buddy. Then his mother, Trish, had been expressing exasperation over the newly acquired puppy, existing out the back of his house. She had suggested bringing him to a shelter in order, perhaps, for them to fix him up with dog training. "He could be an ideal guide dog!" This started Keith thinking and he had said to Peter's dad, upon returning to the house, "What are your feelings as regards matching Peter up with a guide dog? It may allow a significant answer especially if you're considering that wheelchair which I suggested before."

At last, an answer, which in combination would sort out everything? But what was Peter going to think? Yes, he had an opinion and would have to be listened to. When approached, he had initially appeared indifferent. Wishing to assert his position and give himself a worth, he had (as usual) expressed indifference. Pleased that he had been understood to have a worthwhile opinion and having a need to be consulted rather than just being taken for granted.

"A dog is going to be an answer for my sight, he'll be great in my room and I can go no-where! He'll sit in the room and do nothing, great, wonderful. Look I know Dad that you are genuinely concerned and my condition is having a detrimental effect on you and on your life. But what can I do, where can I go? Somehow, somewhere a dog may be an answer but He can't drag me anywhere and I need mobility." Peter had said this and Dad knew the loneliness that he was feeling just by saying it, but now he had an answer. "Suppose that you had that mobility. The answer to you movement was taken care of, would you, now, see the advantage in having a dog, a guide dog? Can you see the advantage in now having both mobility and sight?"

"Perhaps I'm dreaming, but are you suggesting that in one brief moment I can gain both sight and mobility. How? "

"I had planned this as a surprise for you. It was something which I was going to make available to you after appropriate research, but I feel that the time may be appropriate now. So Peter, son, how do you feel about having your very own wheelchair?"

Peter had never considered anything along these lines; he had previously felt that if he would limit himself to a wheelchair, it would be an example of attempting to declare to the world "Hey, look at me, I can do nothing and so feel sorry for me." But the weeks had taken a toll and an imprisonment – although self-imposed, was one which Peter could not determine to be one of an advantage. At last, here was an opportunity for him to break free from his self-appointed isolation and attain his much sought for individualism.

"Of course, there's a lot to be investigated first, before a final selection of a chair is to be decided on. You've kept yourself to yourself for so long that I can understand that this is going to be significant. But I know that, in your hands, the whole plethora of activity will be successful. I want you to leave it in my hands to investigate the whole procedure and I will do the very best for you. I love you and I am going to go forward with you and together we'll rock. Eh?"

Suddenly Peter could begin to understand that a new life was being presented for him to consider. Up until the onset of his own personal illness, he had experienced a form of freedom which was now being denied to him. Within the "rules, boundaries and limitations" of his father's house, he could operate with a degree of freedom.

9. School insistence on a medical examination

He had applied to America for a sports scholarship and got it. The last months had brought about a re-evaluation from him and forced him to concede that life was not going to be quite as sedentary as he might have imagined that it was going to be. He had operated as a partner with Keith (concerning playing soccer) and together they had faced a possible life of athletics and all that that might have involved. Peter's physical condition had suggested that the partnership might no longer be capable of existing but with Dads participation, applications had been made to America.

Peter was applying as an individual with physical concerns (without being exactly specific about his condition). He had been asked at one stage if he used a wheelchair, to which to answered truthfully "No". Given his success on the sports field at home in Ireland and the American wish to promote all things Irish, he had been granted a scholarship. This had also applied to Keith and it further cemented their friendship. Keith was fairly regularly calling to the house with small scraps of inconsequential info, but it kept their friendship alive. Intending to make for America in September, the boys had continued their sport centred lives and it was after one soccer filled afternoon Peter had returned home complaining of headaches (or whatever).

Although it was now the holiday period in Ireland, the two boys were involving themselves in grinds and as a result had to make frequent visits to the school. Soccer was still an integral part of school involvement and the boys were quite unconsciously bonding. Keith had been aware of Peter's complaints, but said nothing, thinking it was only a passing concern. He noticed the deterioration of the physical make-up of his friend and had indeed discussed it with his other friends. The school noticed and some concern was being expressed. But enough was thought to be enough and eventually it was suggested to his parents that a physical examination would be the correct path to go. Peter's record of attendance at school was not the reason for concern, but his physical behaviour and his tolerance to particular physical activity. At times he was noticed to be in a position of appreciating loss of balance and lack of attention. His speech was determined to be deteriorating in presentation – given that he had been a leading light in school debating circles, where his presentation was always considered to be superb.

The school came to understand that no real concern was coming from his home and therefore it was determined to be sensible to request that his parents be summoned to attend a conference within the school. Teachers within Peter's Alma Mater were immediately concerned that their leading star of a pupil was appearing to be slipping to a position of insignificance and mediocrity. What was unknown to the school was that concerning his home life Peter was being recognised as a young man who, for no apparent reason, was exhibiting extreme and serious lack of expected mobility. This lack of mobility had come upon him quite suddenly and with no apparent cause or reason for its existence. It had led his parents to remaining quiet concerning the obvious outcome. His life at home was quite different from what it had been only a very short time before (his parents opinion had been "maybe this will disappear and we'll have our lovely boy back again"). Through discussion and general banter it was proposed by the school that a medical examination might be the appropriate road to go down. The school was anxious to regain their star pupil, whilst the parents were intent on reclaiming their boy back once again.

His G.P. was then approached and Peter's symptoms were revealed for his knowledge. Tests were seen to be gone through and results waited for. The speed of the onset was perplexing and led to an immediate diagnoses not being immediately forthcoming. But with the use of an M.R.I. it became apparent that Multiple Sclerosis may have to be considered as a possible interpretation, or diagnoses.

Single floored existence had been, at home, an immediate solution, which was being lived by Peter. No longer able to, comfortably, negotiate the short flight of stairs up to his first floor bedroom. It had been suggested by his entirely concerned (but confused) father, that one end of the sitting room area be converted to a segregated area for his son. A false wall had been created to allow Peter a degree of privacy and it was this area to which Peter now had reverted – to live in something approximating isolation. He didn't wish to share with anyone and indeed when Keith had called; it was with some reluctance that Peter could tolerate a visit.

Keith had emphasised how at the start of Peter's incapacity, school attendance was still a recognised activity, "but now, Why?" Through the hurt and insignificance Peter had revealed how he had been aware of the total change which he was going to have to bring to his existence. It had been obvious that where only weeks before, people (people in school with him) had actually been looking to him for support and guidance. Now that situation could no longer exist. Indeed, even if he regained all of his previous physicality, memories would remain. No, he had now become a non-person. The only value which he now had was to himself and it was beyond his comprehension how anyone was going to concede that he may have a relative value for anything from this day forward.

10. Discussions between Peter and Keith, Helen and Trish

"**F**eeling sorry for yourself is just the way to go" Keith had responded. "I can understand the way you are feeling, given all that has occurred to you, but DEAL WITH IT. Feeling sorry for yourself is a great way to go – it will lead nowhere. Nothing is going to be gained by this self-centredness. You are being presented with a unique opportunity to turn your life 180 – but no, easier to mull around in self-pity and moroseness. See what you are being given, thank God for it, embrace it and move on."

"This is it! Life gets no better. Sure I'm self-pitying. Why, oh why should I display anything other than total self-pity? You're not the one selected for this special ignominy. Life can be only so cruel and yes, I've copped the lot. In one fell swoop I achieved a hand of cards which make me the luckiest bloke in the world, I don't think so!"

It was with small "tete-a-tete" discourses such as this that the two boys were able to remain on a conversing level of existence, but there were times when Peter was capable of no interaction with another (able bodied individual) and it was then that the relationship between himself and his father would come to the fore. Needing a sounding board of some proportion, he would cry out in a pathetic and self-indulgent fashion. Not giving out to anyone in particular but merely declaring his total frustration at this apparently uncaring world.

But Keith had planted the seeds for a life of purpose and even though Peter had not noticed this subtle infusion, the thought was there; there may be a purpose to all of Peter's indulgences. Something significant could come from this, but it was going to have to be handled in a particular fashion, or form. Enter Max, Dad, Helen and a consortium of circumstances.

The dog had been relegated to a very secondary position (at the back of the house) at this juncture and not a lot of importance was being directed towards him. Trish, hanging the washing out at the start of the day, would periodically trip over him in her endeavours to get to the line. She was, in her own way, concerned for the animal and after a number of encounters had finally considered that with the assistance of the local pound, efforts should come about whereby Max could achieve a practical purpose in his seemingly insignificant life. She consulted with her husband and suggested that with the assistance of the pound, the situation existing at the back of the house could be resolved to every bodies understanding and tolerance. He countered by declaring that the dog was Keith's and that he must be consulted. Being away from the house all day he had no definitive regard for Max and indeed may not at any point in time have remembered his arrival. If the dog was part of the house and he knew nothing about Max then it had to be Keith's concern. Problem over – solved. Keith was questioned by his mother as to his intentions for the Labrador and conceded that at that juncture in time soccer was a more pressing and immediate concern. "Do whatever" and the situation became one of Trish having to entirely work out a course of action.

She had discovered the relevant telephone number whilst engaged at her legitimate employment (in the local library) and shortly it was arranged for Max to be 'rescued'/collected by the same pound and investigations made as to the existence of a suitable training college for training as a guide dog. Speaking to a friend, who also happened to work in the library, she had said as a topic of conversation, that she had just got rid of a dog. The same dog had gone for training as a guide dog but the local pound would have to investigate to find an appropriate training college for him. Throughout continued association and continued interaction, Trish had discovered that Helen (her new friend) had a son who had been recently diagnosed with Multiple Sclerosis and (would you believe it) Helen's son and Trish's son both went to the same school – and they might even know each other.

Well, isn't the world a small place and you never know who it is that you're going to be talking too? Both women had thought that they knew each other and their different circumstances but now, these mutual declarations had served to form a bond of inevitable interaction which dissimilar interests could never have achieved. Further discussion revealed to them both that while Helen had been working away in the library, Trish's son Keith had been calling up most days to visit Helen's son Peter, who had (as already revealed) been recently diagnosed with M.S.. As they had both been involved together in playing soccer and, in point-of-fact, were best friends, this sudden coming together of the mothers should have come about as no surprise.

Helen told Trish (suspecting that it would be confirmed later by Keith) that Peters M.S. was progressive and that although it was particularly debilitating, it was going to get much worse. She was saying this because she had suddenly discovered a mutual point of self-disclosure. She had found someone with whom she could talk and discuss the one principle topic of concern with whom she had found that she could talk with no-one. Dad had been too engrossed with work to ensure that his wife might have someone to share disclosures and concerns with.

No-one else remained to share private sensibilities with and for that reason Helen might have been understood to be similar to a time bomb with her feelings building up within her. Exploding was going to take effect very shortly, but now it seemed that redemption was to hand and a safety valve of words was presenting itself. Thinking that she had known Trish and working with her for a period of years now, she had become settled in a groove of complacency, entirely of her own making. Suddenly it was transpiring that here, within something as inconsequential as a public library, there might exist a form of commonality which had not been known to have existed up until then.

Each woman, centred only upon her own interests, was now being presented with an opportunity to share. This was a condition which had not been understood to have been present before. Demurely the two women approached each other like gladiators, circling around looking for an available opening, only looking for an occasion to meet and share concerns relevant to their immediate mentality.

"Keith has mentioned that he had a friend, who apart from planning to go to America in September with him, was at that moment very sick. But I see so little of him these days (what with soccer and me working in the library) that we could be two different families. Tell me, because I find it strange that we have never got together up until now over this. What are your expectations for the future because I have an idea – with my limited knowledge of MS?"

"Nothing is so bad that it can't get worse. Peter is giving off that his present condition is a mere mishap and displays not being overly concerned. But I think that this is wrong and whatever advantage can be moved towards him, to allow his life to be more tolerable, this then is something that I can only encourage." Helen was close to tears as she sought to bring about this immediate interaction.

Trish was suddenly extremely complacent and wishing to assist in the situation as she understood it to be, coming close to Helen she disclosed that a dog was being given to a pound for movement to a training centre. This dog was going to be trained as a guide dog "and why should Peter not be the one to eventually benefit from the resultant, fully trained dog?"

"If life could only be so simple, Peter has lived in a shell of an existence since he was diagnosed and he goes nowhere. I don't see that a guide dog would be of the slightest support at the moment. What we may be bringing about is a situation where two lives, at least, are entirely messed up, but for your intense concern – thank you".

The tears and compassion between the two women was all which was demonstrating being of concern within the library and the women had to break apart in order to resume work. However, the seeds of something special had been planted, a bond had been created and two people, who may never have come together under different circumstances, were now irreveracobly bound through joint awareness of life with all its foibles.

11. Helen and Dad have conflab

Helen, returning home full of excitement, expecting as it turned out, her husband to be awaiting her. He was behaving as a medical overseer of the mutual concern for them both. Peter was in his area at one end of the sitting room and oblivious to all.

"Darling, something incredible is happening. There is a woman down in the library, who wants to be of help in what we are doing. Sometime ago she gave a dog up to a centre for training as a guide dog. You know that Peter has failing eyesight and it would be brilliant if the two could match up. What do you think?"

Upon consideration, Dad gave out his opinion. "Eyesight is only one consideration for us to be aware of. Guide dogs for Peter would not be of any use whatever within his room. He has to allow himself to leave his space and, to justify the acquisition of a dog; be prepared to open up and face the world on the terms of accepted procedure. He requires mobility, a chance to open up and re-achieve his declared position within that space. As regards the immediate disquiet – mobility, leave that with me and I will work on it, somehow somewhere I have an answer. But again, it will take the approval and support of Peter".

More or less about this time Keith had had his conversation with Dad about the wheelchair and the suggestion that perhaps it might be suitable for Peter to have, as another aid, a guide dog, was going to make the whole arrangement a complete ensemble but Peter had an opinion all of his own and how he would feel about these individual assets were going to have to be considered. Dad could understand that it was not going to be a question of simply taking control of an unknown dog and blasting off with a wheelchair.   Training and familiarisation would have to take effect. Peter?

12. Investigation regarding wheelchairs

A normal wheelchair, if normal could be considered. He knew nothing about what was involved and he knew that it was going to have to be up to him to research the whole plethora of available information. Peter may take his opinions and considerations on board and base his final opinion on what he was able to find out. So he was going to start a progression of finding out information and knowledge of which he had been unaware until now. Time to start........

Going onto the internet he had surfed the respective areas and come up with certain answers. He knew that this would not make him an expert but it would allow him an opinion. He had decided that from the outset he would not allow price to be a determining factor in choosing a wheelchair for his son. A wheelchair being required then a wheelchair was going to become available. He had decided that in order for Peter to feel independent more immediately an electric model was the first consideration. This would result in modifications being made available to the car (for storage) and also having availability to the house and so on.

Peter at this time was not to any degree displaying being paraplegic (or totally incapacitated). Rather he was exhibiting a form of self-pity. He had been told that the condition which was afflicting him was as a result of unknown contributing factors. Then at the time of diagnoses he was told to understand that he was to consider himself dormant. Sure, he was displaying having a myriad of symptoms, but with the diagnoses being unclear and it not being clear that M.S. was the cause of these symptoms, doctors were reluctant to express that M.S. was the disease which was afflicting him. He felt alone and this diagnoses allowed him to withdraw within himself. He was able to talk to his mother and he was telling his friend Keith, who was visiting him every day, but as regards opening up and telling the world, well no, that wasn't a relevant option.

From the onset, loss of balance and loss of vision were symptoms which made it clear that he would have to tell someone who might understand, without being judgemental. The only person who revealed their presence to him, after careful consideration, was his mother. Telling her was both difficult and awkward. He knew nothing of what was occurring to him and he wanted to know why he alone was experiencing what it was that he felt he was suffering. No answers were appearing and his mother told him that she was at much at sea as he was, she didn't understand. She went so far as to suggest that what he might be experiencing might, perhaps, be some sort of growing upset, or illness associated with young men growing older (Peter was 19), but basically she had no idea.

She spoke with her husband who did not initially take the situation seriously. Being involved with an immediate and pressing concern for his company NASA, he said that he did not have the time right then to be dealing with an issue which may resolve itself within a couple of weeks, or whatever. It didn't.

As the first few weeks past and no signs of an improvement were manifesting themselves from Peter, He took a considered step backwards and ever mindful of his family, inquired as to the effect which he could be expected to play in dealing with (what had become now) this family crises. Helen suggested that, given as he was the only one in the family capable of lifting Peter (should it be deemed necessary), it would be advantageous if he would consider remaining at home – for Peter's sake.

His company was consulted and, given his domestic circumstances, they would allow him to operate from home. The bond between himself and Peter grew accordingly and the familiarity between the two reached a new crescendo. Peter was suddenly conceding that within his world was another human being who could (and would) share the hopelessness which he was coming to feel.

Loss of balance, loss of eyesight and a tinkling sensation were working through Peter's body. It was not a voluntary series of feelings which Peter was content with, he hated it and was all the time looking for a reason, an improvement or at least a tangible method with which to deal with this unknown.

Revealing his unwillingness to ascend to his room (and only attempting it when he was certain of no witnesses), it was decided to minimise the sitting room and a dividing wall was set in place. Now he had his own space and God help anyone who encroached onto his space, it was his and he set it up so that all was within his grasp of sight or movement.

Within his room, with no-one to see him, he could indulge in displaying his true feelings. Total despair would settle itself upon this trembling wreck of a body, which was what he imagined was all that was left to him. There was no improvement that was going to visit itself upon him (subconsciously he would not have allowed it). He had been dealt a particular hand of cards by life and he was stuck with them. A recovery was not going to come about and therefore "let's feel sorry for ourselves".

Permanent patient always getting worse, oh dear! No more this vital, needed, required individual who was always to the fore in everything. This essential 19 year old, who had always been known to lead the way; the first into everything, was now having to concede that the consequences were there to be dealt with by someone else. By saying all this, it is being seen that Peter was quite unprepared to take the part of a follower and indeed to his thinking it was always essential to be out in the front and seen to be there.

Having suddenly, managed to attain this unwanted plethora of physical symptoms/characteristics and having been thrust into this miss-mash of contentious capabilities, resignation was all which appeared available to him – despair! His world was reduced, to those people whom he could expect to have interaction with, through necessity. Fortunately this consisted of a world of three people. His father, mother and a close friend who he was being expected to hit The States with, all things allowing him to do so.

His father had encouraged him and made it possible for him in the very early stages of his diagnoses, to seek an athletic scholarship from a faculty in America. He was coming to the end of his assumed school career and was not displaying having any further ambitions. With his father's assistance and indeed support, he sought academic continuance in The States. As Dad was an extremely well-regarded employee within NASA, acquisition of the scholarship had turned out to be no problem at all and Peter's expectation of further education was a foregone conclusion. He had applied for enrolment at the very start of his M.S. involvement and therefore did not have too much to disclose (in all honesty) to the academic authorities. He had however requested one consideration. Having revealed (by letter) that he had had no experience of being away from home and therefore might display tendencies towards homesickness, he had requested that his friend Keith accompany him, should he be successful.

Where Peter had always graduated towards the position of being captain of whatever team he had been contracted to join, Keith was recognised to always be the side-kick. Ever there to support in whatever way, his approved and leading partner, Peter and Keith became known as a 'pair of Siamese Twins', where one went the other was always found. Ultimately Keith was also successful in his application to take advantage of an American scholarship, within the one university as his friend Peter

At that stage M.S. had made a significant intrusion into the expected progress of life for the two eager and intelligent youths. Almost (or so it seemed) week by week further levels of disability were manifesting themselves for Peter to contend with. He was finding it awkward to maintain balance, his available eyesight was deteriorating and he was aware (within himself) of uncontrollable shakes. He started to withdraw. He broke association with friends; he almost had nothing to say to his family and appeared to be taking his condition for himself, on himself, with no tangible regard for anyone. Slowly he came to allow himself to feel that at this stage life was dealing him a hand of cards which (regardless of his own personal feelings) was a hand which he was just going to have to accept and deal with, neither knowing the game or the rules. In a twisted and perverse way "Hell, it was all fun, I think not.

Meanwhile Dad was resigning himself to finding out all about wheelchairs. From the start, he hadn't known much. Indeed if it is a subject with which one is unacquainted, why bother? From the start he came to appreciate the number of different types and models (one size not fitting all). The most basic and accepted type was the manual. Thinking of wheelchairs in general, this is the one which comes immediately to mind. A development from this is the electric and it was in this direction that he was being drawn.

Dad didn't look forward to his son reverting to an existence in a wheelchair but he was realistic enough to see that this was the direction in which Peter was going and if that was the way in which it was going to be, well let's make it as easy as possible.

Throughout these deliberations the medical assessments were always on-going and it was at the various locations for examination that Peter had been able (not with any great enthusiasm) to receive an introduction to the phenomena of wheelchairs. Initially he had stumbled along various pathways, in order to get to rooms of investigation. But this was seen to be too slow and Dad had resorted to assisting him. Finally a wheelchair was suggested and everyone was left wondering why this had not been thought of at the very beginning.

It had not grabbed Peter as being a particularly clever way to go. The wheelchair was too stiff and ungainly to steer, as if in an expected fashion for an athlete. But with practice he appeared to develop a technique of his own and had almost begun to look forward to his hospital visits in order to refine and perfect his individualism for chair control.

Things at this stage were now becoming critical and it was proposed that Keith head off for America alone, leaving Peter to understand that a stabilizing of his condition could be expected fairly shortly and if things were then becoming tolerable (if ever!) he would join Keith and resume some sort of life.

In America Keith could press on and discover how life was to be run and by the time Peter was going to join him, he could be expected to know the ruses to pull in order to enjoy life as a student. Keith had all but forgotten Max, at this juncture and it was Trish who was acting as the go-between as regards Max's integration with the training facility and would-be proposed patients. Bill had been looking to send Max back to where he had come from, but the pound dismissed the return by stating that Max had not been their responsibility but instead had come from Keith's house. Bill, on an extremely unofficial turn from protocol had come to be aware of the existence of Keith's home and had gone round to it to achieve some sort of understanding as regards Max.

It was at this time that Trish had suggested Peter, as a prospective and suitable recipient for Max. Helen had sort of approved her suggestion and it having been said it was left, for the moment, in that state of flux. Bill could only keep Max at the facility for so long; Trish had an inherent fear about resuming responsibility for Max and it looked as though it was all going to be dependent on Peter.

Diminishing eyesight, lack of apparent mobility, residual shakes, and loss of focus, minimal concentration and various other manifesting conditions were now making themselves an appreciated and integral part of the person whom Peter could now only recognise as himself.

Suddenly Dad was going to bring about a solution to difficulties perceived within this scenario. He was proposing that a wheelchair and a dog could be the answer, taken together; they could be understood to provide both desired mobility and sight for Peter.

13. Miraculous Healing

At this point in time a friend of the family (he was mentioned before), Tim had suggested something for Peter to consider. Tim was a realist and not contemptuously noted for pragmatic opinions on what he was just then going to accept that Peter was to ponder.

"Religion"!

Tim had this ability to throw in one word invectives, accepting that this would cover everything. Peter, far from dismissing this proposal, wanted to take it further, if only to allow Tim to know that his single word monologues were not something to be seen as worthy of attention. "So let's allow Tim to lengthen his motion and come to concede that it truly is ridiculous."

Turning to Tim, Peter asked him to elaborate.

"Well I know so little about it, myself. But I am aware that between yourself and your dad you may have exhausted all rational, realistic paths for helping someone in your condition. I suggest that you now investigate the where-with-all of 'divine assistance'. Your own personal opinion may be one of pooh-poohing the entire notion, but allow yourself to accept that there is more to life then we can fully comprehend at the moment and what we don't understand now we can know as being termed supernatural. I know that there is existing, now, a cure for your condition. But as human beings we are unaware of it. However as a result of a greater power/force making us appreciate, outside of our subjective understanding, that a solution to whatever is available and we only have to accept it, in order to benefit as regards a benevolent outcome, a miraculous answer may be awaiting you".

This timely conjecture by Tim initially perplexed Peter, it was only some time later that he resolved to take it further and investigate. Alone in his room, where he had access to the most up to date computer data (Dad being an I.T. wizard), he perused the internet. He looked up such things as Miraculous Healing and was initially fascinated by disclosures such as a revelation that one source of miraculous healing appears to emanate from a religious grotto at a place called Lourdes.

This is in the southern reaches of France (the Pyrenees) and the story goes that in the mid 1800's a young girl saw an apparition of the Virgin Mary. She was told to drink from a well, which had 'miraculously' appeared just in front of her. The first accredited miracle associated with this well was in 1858 and since then it has been conceded that up to 60 miracle healings have occurred.

Peter, initially, thought that his requirements could be about to be resolved from this same grotto, he was excited. The next day, in conversation with Dad, he disclosed his wish to take this further and make available the benefits of Lourdes. His Father, ever the pragmatist, immediately conceded that his son was now in need of psychiatric help and physical assistance which would require the support of mental assistance and could perhaps lead to a situation where an answer might become available.

"What have I ever done to allow you to see any truth in Christian dogma? I'm telling you, all you are going to discover is a bunch of superstitious, blinded, controlled and manipulating hypocrites".

Peter started to cry, the tears coming from some suppressed memory which allowed him to remember a time when it had been normal for him to walk, to talk, to perform such basic functions as going to the toilet – by himself. Now all that had been taken away and in its place – this dependency, this hopelessness and this need to involve other people in everything he was doing.

But now, this temptation; this call to correct the standard of life which he had been thrust into, a glorious reawakening; being hindered by his father and reinforced by his not knowing.

Yes, the Church was a mystery, but only because he had been brought up to live in a world of physics and mathematics. Where there was a reason and a cause for everything. Mystery only existed in order to be explained and then understood. The strength of the church lay in the mystery it evoked; claiming direct interaction with an invisible force called God. Worked by men having power (authority) over other men, because God said so!

But if this dogma, this theology, could bring about a reverse of the situation in which he now found himself; should he not then be a supporter of this new-found truth, it being more relevant and true for him. He told his father that he understood the pertinent reasons for his lack of faith (if it mattered) but this revelation, being disclosed to him, was just too big, too much needing to be investigated, just to be ignored.

He cried, yes, it was entirely from self-pity, he wanted the life which he had once had back again. He told his father that he was going to investigate The Church and that it would be an investigation incorporating no mumbo-jumbo, no unrealistic high-brow anathema which could only lead to ultimate confusion. He was going to approach his investigation as he had learnt to deal with all concerns – with tolerance and diligence. At 19 years of age, it was time for him to strike out and claim an understanding of what was truth (to him).

In this time, this age, he didn't need to even leave his room. All answers would come to him. He wasn't one of these computer junkies, those mindless clowns who could sit for hours pushing buttons with nothing achieved after hours of 'play' except a score of unrelated intensity; these empty brains with nothing to show except a litany for their own self-justifying immaturity and incompetence. Surfing the net had been an occupation of his, true, but only in a quest to gain a better understanding of a particular concern – he had wanted information.

Now he would use the internet to investigate The Church. He thought about procedure, protocol and then he acted. He had, in his mind, been drawn towards Lourdes and on the internet he sought out a relevant map. He opened up what he was seeing and came to understand that what he was looking at was the grotto within this location. He understood that his father was regarding him with curiosity, but saying nothing. With intensity he leaned in close to the screen and opened up a 3D appreciation. He was conscious of discordant colours appearing at either end of the same grotto and presenting confusing colour above walkways leading to and from the said grotto. He brought in his vision and suddenly understood that what he was looking at was lines of unattended crutches. These were un-needed accomplices for people who had approached the grotto for a healing and as a direct result of a healing having been achieved; the related crutch was a no longer needed appendage. In gratitude they had been left at the point of their last being needed. Like solitary sentinels they stood silently to attention, waiting for nothing, a silent reminder to a time of integrity and usefulness, when their very existence had determined the capability of the incumbent and relevant owner. Here was an indelible sign that something was working, a portrayal from the Church, an undisclosed statement saying in a hushed and muted voice that immediately before their incarceration in their presented position, a miracle of healing had occurred.

Peter, fraught with intensity and awareness, continually muttered to himself "and still there is no sign. I see what is being shown to me but in this regard and pertaining to what has happened I concede that there must be more". He scrolled along the path, coming to a pile of loosely gathered crutches; he paused at the map disclosures and carefully examined what he was seeing.

His intense attention and overall concern registered interest from his father. Dad leaned forward and inquired in a desultory manner as to the source of Peter's concern.

"I've been brought to this stage of appreciating validity by recognising all which I can see; finding what I am looking for will permit me to take this Miracle Healing to a position of conceding it to actually be true and available. I just have to satisfy myself as to the existence of an extraneous point. One which will satisfy not only yourself but the whole argument as to the entire question of miracle healing but I don't see what I am looking for yet".

On his computer screen he moved nearer to the grotto, finally coming to a halt at the end of the line of crutches. His vision closed in and he surveyed all which was available for him to see. He leaned back in the chair and with resignation he declared "And not one prosthesis. All of the line shows crutches. People having the physical requirements to walk – legs! But no-where is displayed the earth shattering existence of the miracle of having no propensity for being able to walk and the sudden acquisition of a pair of legs – or even one. This confirms the argument for a situation of mind over matter and not a convincing appraisal for the existence of a God".

"What is being displayed here is a very limiting portrayal of a particularly weak God. The Church has seen fit to present an image of a very mediocre example of apparent divine intervention and has missed the opportunity of displaying a beyond refuting example of a Miracle. Crutches support a body with the attributes of an ability to walk. Prosthesis, lying against the wall, would reveal, to all, the occurrence of taking a person with the physical capability of not being able to walk – no leg and immediately bestowing upon the incumbent the required physical status of a biped. Now that would be an undisputed Miracle".

"I am being shown a particularly inane and forced disclosure of a human attempt at forcing an infantile and initially spectacular existence of a power with no power. It's in the mind and those bodies who have approved the leaving behind and displaying of redundant crutches are missing the very next persuasive tool; the displaying of a prosthetic limb".

Now beyond conjecture, that would open up to world attention the actual existence of a power unknown and not understood. But no, no evidence of a happening other than complete mind control. You (the individual) are told that a miracle *may* be available, believe all that I'm telling you and 'spontaneous' benefits will occur. The mind is infused with the possibility of an actual happening and the groundwork is being laid whereby the happening emanates from the body of the individual. A healing comes about (a spectacular and wonderful occurrence- a miracle) and in gratitude crutches are laid along the wall. But no prosthesis has ever revealed itself to be amongst the displayed. Can there be a credible reason? Let's go to the top.

Individuals have made this a club of their own, with rules and guidance brought about by themselves for adherence by lesser beings within the club. "I am a mangled person, seeking a cure for what is a life changing condition and in order to avail of a miraculous spontaneous cure; I have to adhere to all the dictates of this prescribed club. All that I can conclude is 'maybe not so'".

Through-out this diatribe, Dad had forced himself into a position of being a spectator. He had instilled within his son a particular way of addressing life. Questioning it to a particular understanding and now he would be seeing the outcome of his upbringing upon his immediate progeny. Peter, to an understanding, had sized up the pro-offered institution of the Church. He had sensed a flaw in the presented picture and based on that had confined himself to a decision. Peter conceded that Faith Healing may be an actuality but the human capability of perusing proof; well it left a desire for further annunciation.

Peter had had his expectations of Miraculous Healings sorely upset. He had to broaden his outreach and consider a more fundamental and physical means of procuring his much sought after healing. Now he was in the possession of a wheelchair and a dog. He had to consider putting them together. He decided that with Keith now in America, Mum (Helen) now working satisfactory hours in the library and Dad creating as many hours as possible, at home – to work, he would take off around the county. He would reveal to himself the capabilities of both the Chair and the Dog. It would necessitate the understanding of using public transport and accessibility for his Wheelchair, but he knew this would all be within his scope and grasp.

14. Kilmuckridge

He first of all would decide on a forthcoming destination. He settled on a picturesque beach, in County Wexford, by the name of Kilmuckridge. But to get there was going to necessitate his sense of individuality coming to the fore by determining his immediate form for travelling. The opportunity was there to avail of public transport, so he proposed reviewing everything involved accordingly. He investigated (by telephone) the times and procedures of taking a bus from where he was, to get too Kilmuckridge.

He faced an initial problem. He had to understand that as far as Irish society was concerned he was different and as much as Irish society cried out claiming to wish to better the Irish segment of their society which was experiencing a disability, I think not. The leading transport concern for the country was an outfit called Bus Eireann and they were not immediately disposed to be helpful towards someone experiencing physical attributes similar to those which Peter was revealing.

He revealed a wish to have wheelchair access ability for himself. Down the road this was available should he be travelling from Dublin, Waterford, Cork or Galway. But from such a minor concern as his hometown to Kilmuckridge, no go. But being fair to Bus Eireann, They were increasing the number of their selected wheelchair assisted locations with a propensity which was going to be astounding. But it would be a question of taking them at their time and meanwhile relaxing in a wheelchair waiting. God Almighty! If just one, just one of the hierarchal clowns sitting in an office, kitted out with daily requirements - access to a gymnasium, coffee machine and ease of movement to their associates or friends, if just one of these bureaucrats could change places with someone reliant on decisions made by them for even one day, how different life would be for the handicapped in our society. But no and so we sit and wait.

It was going to be necessary to plan ahead. Notification to the authorities of an intended bus journey, complete with wheelchair, involved the need to remove four seats from the bus. So society can realise that a commercial outfit (such as a bus company) might be reluctant to reduce the number of seats available for paying customers and be reluctant to make way for wheelchair assisted passengers. Did anyone ever question a single wheelchair user in order to find out their willingness in accepting their condition?

A particular lift (or hoist) was needed to bring the chair up from the pavement on to the bus in question. Small mannerisms such as this were being used to reveal to the world, how different and debilitating wheelchair users could become. Perhaps it would be better to just ignore them. Perhaps they might kindly fade away. If we don't (or can't) see them, maybe we can imagine that these subjugated people are not, to any degree there, to be even considered.

Peter investigated all that there was to investigate as far as making a Bus available for himself. It was a pointless task and only emphasised to him how society was being geared to the able-bodied and the whole. His father stepped in and explained that the situation being what it was maybe a taxi or mini-bus could be an answer. He understood that he would be too involved, with work at home, to be in a position to render physical (present) assistance to his son at chosen locations – even though they may be close to home. He also understood his son's desire for relative independence. Peter would do this by himself.

Early in his life, Peter and The Clan (as he unambiguously referred to his family) had partaken of a holiday in Kilmuckridge and it had left an indelible mark or memory on Peter. He wished to re-achieve that feeling of personal empowerment which his early days had allowed him.

In order to claim and regain this memory he would have to get down there and indeed having got there he would have to allow himself to have a reason to be there. An immature and insidious reason such as a regained holiday location memory from the time of his youth would not be a sufficient reason, so he elected to go to this holiday area and investigate available gems of information. Indeed he decided to make this his justifying reason to go wherever. He conceded that his arc of available movement may be his chair and with diminishing eyesight the aural disclosures pertaining to the area may be sufficient.

His father understood the difficulties that Peter was going through in order to simply obtain passage to a single location. He appreciated the obstacles presenting themselves in order for his son to allow his life to continue in such a way as to allow him to feel a useful person within his society. So he suggested to Peter that they make use of a friend and avail of a local taxi service.

Dave was a next-door neighbour and a driver with a local taxi company. He immediately stepped up to the mark and was available to convey wherever. Now Max had to be considered. Having only recently come under the tutelage of Peter, Dave wanted to know that Max was going to behave with appropriate and correct behaviour; as regards travelling within a car or minibus. Peter gave assurances that as Max was a potentially fully trained guide dog, no upset would be expected or tolerated. So all seemed to be coming together and Kilmuckridge was drawing closer.

It wasn't a particularly long journey and it was decided that a Minibus would be the most suitable form of conveyance. Dave could choose between Minibus and car. So on the day selected Peter was outside the house waiting for Dave to arrive, in order to pick himself and Max up. His mother, Helen, was working in the library at the time but his father broke away from whatever he was doing and was waiting to bid Peter adieu.

It was a sunny day and all appeared well for the proposed excursion. Dave arrived and after some unfamiliarity as regards loading and securing (Dave explaining the intricacies), they set off. Kilmuckridge, as far as travelling by minibus was concerned, was only a short distance and the journey was completed relatively quickly. Peter had asked to be dropped outside of the Londis supermarket – from where he felt that all things which he required were within reach. Dave deposited him in the expected place and then left.

The significance of the moment filtered in through Peter's psyche and he leant forward to where Max was sitting (being ever attendant to his handler's intentions). He caressed the dog's ears and declared that to all understanding the world was now theirs. Feeling that what was going to be important was what was going to be said, rather than picturesque post card scenery, Peter turned his wheelchair towards Ned Kavanagh's house. The dog reacted in sync and appeared to lead the way, ever attentive for further instructions other than Peter giving him the initial "Forward".

Back at home, on the internet, Peter had investigated Kilmuckridge and seen that a local celebrity (or historian) had been given out as being called Ned Kavanagh. He was a published author and indeed Peter had even downloaded some of his pro-offerings. He thought that if he might ever get the chance to meet him, Peter could get a stock of information concerning Kilmuckridge from this one source.

He knew the way to his house; by having uploaded Ned's address (contact details at the back of a particular book) onto his computer; he had appreciated the way to Ned's house through disclosures from the 3D internet map. Moments later he arrived, to be met by three dogs on the veranda of an extension by the side of a house. He knew he was in the right area because of a van parked outside with Ned Kavanagh's name on the side of it.

A gentle man with a flowing beard greeted Peter, tall and with a nautical gait (belying his land-based working activities}. He enthusiastically welcomed Peter to his home, asking in what connection he had deserved this visitation. Peter responded by disclosing that he had become aware of Ned and his existence in relation to being in a position to reveal pertinent facts concerning Kilmuckridge. As an incumbent with the condition of Multiple Sclerosis, Peter asked for Ned's understanding and forbearance in relation to his obvious physical limitations.

As Peter would obviously not be able to actively partake in the obvious and immediate advantages of the pro-offered Kilmuckridge rural scenario, he hoped that Ned would allow him an insight into gems of useful historical interest concerning the area. Having immediate sympathy for Peter and his obvious incapacities, Ned assured the same that such as his knowledge would allow, would be Peter's for the asking.

Peter was aware that all the planning and activity relating to his actually being able to get down to Kilmuckridge, meant that his visit was going to be brief and immediate. He wouldn't have a great deal of time to share a physical interaction with Ned so salutations having been conducted he awaited for what Ned was going to disclose.

15. The kill 'em and eat 'ems

"As you've said; there's not a lot of point in telling you of the holiday sights and activities of the surrounding area, so instead I am going to tell you of a gem of information of which few people may be aware. A long time ago and not so far away, and it was at a time when the weather was at its worst, individuals were intent on the procuring of certain apparently unobtainable goods; for their own benefit. To do so they used to involve themselves in the securing of ancient storm lanterns to a single one of their cows out on the beach above the storm tossed seas. Mariners close in to the treacherous coastline would be fooled into thinking that the permitted light was a light coming from a lighthouse somewhere within the vicinity. They would make navigational errors resulting in the floundering of the same vessel, which would then be seized upon by the local insurgents and stripped of all required desired commodities.

Right, well there was one time; I think the year was 1766 and the ship in question was going by the name of The Welcome.

The night was particularly rough and a group of neer-do-wells were assembled on the beach (just off from Kilmuckridge/Morriscastle). Gain was within their minds when they spied a luckless vessel bearing down along the Wexford coast. Seizing a hapless cow and securing a lantern to its horns, they waited in the dark night for whatever was going to transpire. The ship floundered on the adjacent sandbar and the surviving sailors weakened and eventually making their way onto the shore were seized upon and seeing such appendages as the rings on the unfortunates hands, the sailors were killed and the locals in their absolute poverty were driven to gnaw the fingers of the dead mariners to make the rings their own.   Rumour has it that the coastguard of the day was shortly in attendance and getting on board the same vessel, shouted out "anyone on board", a parrot up in the mast area answered, "They killed 'em and they ate 'em ".   So was brought into existence the reference to 'the kill 'ems and eat 'ems' of the local area. A final peculiarity to the story is that the ship was supposed to have been owned by the nuns, operating from somewhere within the Wexford area. A possible truth to this story is that the ship may, in fact, have been owned by merchants by the name of Nunne. Such is the seriousness and depth of belief in local gossip and rumour. Look, I can stand here and gossip with you about revelations concerning the lands of Kilmuckridge/Morriscastle but not a lot will be achieved so I will leave it at that for the moment – as I've got things to be doing and some place to go. If you are genuinely interested in pursuing a working knowledge of the area, I suggest the involvement of libraries and books. Should you require my assistance in the future please do not hesitate to seek me out? Now I noticed that when you arrived at my house, your dog did not react with either of my spaniels? Given the available Kilmuckridge mentality of being open and welcoming to all strangers, can you explain"?

Peter retorted by disclosing that Max was a guide dog and that therefore he was totally amenable to all creatures which he may encounter on his daily walks, so Ned should not be in the slightest surprised or concerned with the reaction which he had seen displayed. Max was contentedly surveying all that was his wont to revue.   His charge (and responsibility) was ever present and contentedly instructing him in the way in which he should always present himself – no need for concern. He prepared to leave, being aware that Peter was close to concluding business with Ned.

Upon Peter having concurred with Ned as to his amenability to receive phone calls in the future (in order to maintain a line of contact), the instruction "Forward" came and Max (ever compliant) sprang forward, away from the house and intent on assuming further adventures of which he would have no idea. Peter directing the electric wheelchair and assuming a position to the rear of Max proceeded back to the Londis area of Kilmuckridge.

Arriving back at the supermarket forecourt, Peter (looking around) was aware of a man approaching him from the direction of the front door of the same supermarket. Being unable to detect any certain details (because of diminishing eyesight) Peter was cognisant of the individual approaching him with the intention of sharing familiarities with Max. Peter disclosed in the direction of the aforementioned man that Max was a working guide dog and that he should be approached, or considered, as being an integral part of Peter with his wheelchair. He was a work in progress and therefore ought not to be fraternised with.

Lowering a clip-board, Hugh (the manager of the supermarket) having changed his mind from approaching Max, revealed an intention to instead converse with Peter. Not recognising Peter as a local and for the purposes of promotion of his supermarket, he inquired as to Peter's purpose for being in the locality. Peter (ever anxious to boost his own image) replied that he had gained a scholarship to an American University and having sent a partner over to the States in order to check out disability conditions therein, was engaged in using available time – before he might go across himself, to gain an understanding of his own locality. Knowing that Ned Kavanagh may have a certain standing to the knowledge of this man, now in front of him, he revealed that he had just come from Ned and that he was intent on furthering his knowledge of the Kilmuckridge area.

The man laughed and introduced himself as Hugh Corrigan – the manager of the supermarket which they were now outside of. He expressed initial interest in the dog beside the wheelchair, declaring himself to be a lover of animals. How he had appreciated the obvious bond between dog and handler. If indeed he could be of assistance to Peter, in his quest for knowledge concerning the immediate area, then Hugh would make himself available.

It was Peters turn to laugh and he replied by disclosing that people were coming to the fore, Ned and himself were the first two people whom he had encountered in Kilmuckridge and that they had both suggested disclosing of pertinent facts concerning the area. His task of investigation may be, now, one of particular ease and that the Kilmuckridge area may now not be as stupefying as had once appeared. People were allowing themselves to be of assistance in dealing with another human being whereas corporate bodies could effectively hid behind their façade of cold and unfeeling indifference.

Hugh countered by suggesting (to Peter's surprise) that they weren't even standing on Kilmuckridge soil. "I understand that you may not be in a position to follow my disclosures quite as intently as might be appropriate but", moving away from the supermarket entrance and looking down the road towards Blackwater, "you may be able to see the horizon down towards the south. Just under the horizon there is a graveyard and that marks the extent of the original northern boundary of the original Kilmuckridge. Far from being an expert on the matter, I am at least somewhat aware of the entire situation. It would appear that originally the post office for the village of Kilmuckridge was in the house just opposite to the Protestant cemetery. It moved to a position just across the road from this supermarket and remained there for some time (outside the original limits of the village). The area of the new position was called Litter, with the name of the immediate area being referred to as The Ford. On relevant Electoral Rolls for this area, the location is still named as The Ford and, as I said, the limits of Kilmuckridge end at the cemetery. All of this area, from here as far as Blackwater (heading south) and over towards Morriscastle, or even on northwards towards Ballygarret is overflowing with history and I would think that you could gain enough knowledge to very easily write a book, if you do, don't forget where the original idea came from, hint-hint ya!"

Peter was exceptionally grateful for this new information and felt that he may now be in receipt of knowledge of which the average person may not actually be aware. This was going to put him in a very invidious position as regards having intimate knowledge concerning areas of which he was going to be conducting investigations. His next location for investigation was Enniscorthy Castle.

16. Enniscorthy

Living in the south-east of Ireland, Enniscorthy was no stranger to Peter and he knew that going into Enniscorthy would be no challenge to him. Now, however he would be going in armed with an Electric Wheelchair and a Guide dog. He speculated that he may find it more or less friendly to negotiate. Time was going to tell. Dave (his minibus driver) had exchanged conversation with Peter and it was agreed that Dave would deposit Peter at a significant location suitable for the wheelchair bound incumbent. He would leave Peter at a place called Treacy's Hotel. This was in the area (or so he knew it to be) close to the castle. Peter was accompanied by Max and felt that it would be more appropriate to follow pedestrian crossings in order to make his way from the hotel and up to the castle.

Dave had alerted a receptionist as to Peters' presence outside the hotel and the receptionist had asked Peter if he wished to go immediately to the castle or would he like to partake of a beverage. Peter elected to partake of a cup of coffee and with Max acting as his eyes; he gained entry to the hotel by an entrance door (wheelchair accessible) to the left of the main door. Making their way through a dining area, they made their way past the toilets and came into a bar area. Peter turned his chair towards a table and with Max lying down in front of the chair, he awaited his coffee. He looked around and detecting shapes – rather than forms, he sought to enter a conversation with a person sitting over beside the bar.

The person understood that Peter had diminished eyesight and introduced himself as Sam. He enquired as to how debilitated Peter was. Peter revealed that he had M.S. and that it had been diagnosed as progressive. His eyesight was the one factor which was concerning him the most. Although it was getting worse, it had not reached a stage of leaving him completely blind, just yet, but now he found himself having to do a double take for everything. He could detect the fact that it was now becoming noticeably more obvious that he had become much more dependent on such tools as his chair and his dog. He was aware that his ability to walk, to any degree, was now gone and that as a result his chair was his only means of effective movement.

The coffee had arrived and with the aid of a straw, Peter was able to partake of the same. There was a small rack which could be brought to the front of Peters chair and lowered into position, in order to support a cup. With a lid on the top of the cup and with a hole in the centre supporting a straw, drinking could commence. Between conversing with his new acquaintance and drinking his coffee, Peter almost forgot what the purpose of his being in Enniscorthy was in the first place. He reached down to where he knew Max to be and finding the dog, he stroked his ear. He finished his coffee and being led by the dog, returned to the street the way he had come. He was aware that the traffic was going to present a problem for him, at that stage and with the entire movement passing in front of his eyes he knew that the traffic was reasonably heavy.

Knowing of the required pedestrian crossing, he instructed Max to lead in the direction of it. Max approached the crossing and sat down – awaiting further instructions. Looking both ways and being aware of a relevant gap in vehicular movement, Max stood. The cars approaching the crossing had now come to a halt, permitting the incumbent in the wheelchair, time to cross the road. Hearing no moving traffic, Peter called for Max to lead across "Forward". Max moved, being closely followed by the wheelchair.

They crossed the road and moved down towards the bridge. The occasional pedestrian passed them, leaving plenty of room for the wheelchair to proceed. The walkway narrowed and it soon became obvious that the wheelchair was going to take up the entire available space. Mutterings were heard concerning the obvious nuisance value of people in wheelchairs, whilst the same individuals stepped into the roadway hoping that drivers of cars bearing down on them would appreciate the pedestrians' presence on the same roadway. Never a one to ask if the wheelchair user was occupying his chair out of choice, as if it were perfectly understandable that fully mobile and agile persons would break from their customary habit of perambulation and instead resort to inconveniencing society by taking up all available space on whatever pathway, in the same wheelchairs. It was made more difficult by Peter not even being able to look the oncoming pedestrian in the eye; in order to make his excuses and thereby bring into existence some sort of understanding (he cursed his diminishing eyesight).

Together, dog and wheelchair incarcerate began to cross the bridge and (from memory) Peter knew that the castle lay a short distance across the road. In vain he looked at the surface of the road. His eyesight would not allow him to distinguish individual faces or particular detail of everyday life, but he knew that a pedestrian crossing was quite distinguishable and he thought that he really ought to be able to make such a thing out, but no, a single monotone appreciation came to him. A tone which revealed an undisturbed road surface such as was all that was apparent to him, looking with his undistinguishing eyes.

All that he had to do now was attain a crossing of this one road, here in front of him (the N11), but with traffic showing an intention to alter, on a permanent basis, the physical makeup of any unthinking person who would venture away from the safety offered by the walkway, he felt no such inclination. He knew that the castle lay to his front and secretly wished that months earlier he might have familiarized himself with the whereabouts of relevant pedestrian crossings in a town so close to his actual home.

Max was not a great asset in these circumstances and with traffic pouring down, on a continual basis; there was no chance that Max was going to lead his handler in crossing the N11. Peter knew that he had left a pedestrian crossing, behind him at Treacys Hotel and simple intelligence told him that if he went up the road (towards Dublin) he was going to eventually find an elusive crossing that would take him across the road to where he wished to go. He directed Max to continue on their walk away from Treacys, knowing that success would eventually be theirs. But before the pair left the western end of the older bridge crossing the Slaney, Peter cast a final unseeing eye across the road and remembered a time when that piece of road could have seemed like a friend, a shortcut on his intended path to wherever he was going to go.

Together they moved off, Max on the left hand side and Peter bearing the consequences of the pervading surface. Moving away from the bridge, the incumbent in the wheelchair now thought of intended possibilities, he knew that in his vicinity, on a week day (this was Saturday) he could have expected a seemingly divine answer to his inherent concern. A Lollipop Man, of distinction, as he remembered it, by the name of Eamon Sheridan was in place to assist schoolgoers in their attempts at crossing the road. As it was a day outside of his working week – no Eamon. He had heard it said (amongst his friends' months earlier) how Enniscorthy was suggesting its tolerance towards wheelchairs and their occupants. He thought how, apart from anything else, it showed that the governing entities of the town might be considered to at least have a sense of humour.

Whatever sight remained with him was trained intently on the northward winding N11. He knew that between where they were and the outer limits of the town, somewhere, there must lie this required pedestrian crossing. Bureaucratic demeanour could not surely allow a wheelchair user to find their way to where he was and have to remain there. Max led on.

His mobile rang with his mother seeking his attention. She had rung – from the library (during a break) and being aware of his proposed adventure in the town, was ringing to inquire as to his achieved success. He mentally strengthened himself. Looking in the direction of the dog, he bit his cheek and responded by suggesting that everything was in hand and going just how he had foreseen that it would. He was close to his mother and it didn't sit well with him that he couldn't (or wouldn't) break down, as he felt that he wanted to ask for her help and remain where he was until she could come to where he was and help. In his mind he was telling himself that he was nineteen and now a young man, he ought to be able to cope and this was just such an occasion whereby he might just demonstrate making a stand for himself, he would do it, he could do it. Yes mother dear, he was AOK and pushing on with his chosen individual task. She hung up and Peter was left with a feeling of being entirely on his own.

He felt that he had covered about a quarter of a kilometre and that something should be revealing itself. He had traversed a large number of different walkway surfaces and considered with disinterest the road to his left. He knew of the surface that had been applied less than a year before. How he had joked with his friends of how this resurfacing would allow them to nearly kill themselves, in times to come, when each one of them would be travelling that same stretch with girlfriends and showing off.

Someone came out of a commercial concern on their right hand side and after apologising for getting in the way enquired if all was okay. Peter broke out of his melancholy demeanour and suggested that if the person, whom he had just met, was involved in business this far out of town then he must be involved in something very particular. He was told that the place which the person had just come from was called L.M. motors and that he had just been engaged in a conversation concerning parking the car which was being left in for servicing. It seemed to be that there was limited parking within the garage forecourt and it had not been allowed, by the authorities, to park surplus cars, relating to the garage, immediately outside the forecourt along the N11. This was contentious because on the far side of the road and nearer to the town, there was a large supermarket. This same supermarket was allowed and indeed did on frequent occasions block the entire N11 in order to allow the delivering Lorries access to the related loading bays; for deliveries. It appeared that money had a way of talking and with money came power. Authority might have a need for the little man, in the general scheme of things, but let's not reveal being helpful. As a result society would allow opportunities to go in the direction of the big guns, the interests with money, but "let's tolerate the little man and keep him in his place". The little man might contribute but let's be modern and realistic.

Peter could hear, in his mind, the rhumbunciousness of city councillors as they strove to justify their individual position on whatever council. Not anymore the need for integrity or the pursuance and completion of their plaintiff pleas on the canvass trail. Having been selected to occupy a position of power, were they just acting in order to promote their name?

He; stuck in a wheelchair, needing a pedestrian crossing, was dependant on the benevolence of city tsars, to effect a bestowal of urban funds for the purpose of simply crossing the road and resuming a journey of integral value. Thoughts tormented him of all his previous concerns and acquaintances. He pitied himself and centred on that awareness failed to grasp a broader picture. He was as guilty of self-interest as the pundits whom he was seeking to make responsible.

He asked, in hopelessness, the person coming away from L and M motors, if they were aware of a relevant pedestrian crossing which would take him across the road. The person laughed and then appreciating (in embarrassment) Peters' predicament as regards eyesight, he looked up the N11 away from the garage and said, "Well in all my time dealing in this garage, I've never had to worry about crossing the road in order to get to the sales area on the far side. Literally yards up the N11 (beside the garage) there is in fact what you're looking for; a crossing and it comes with lights etcetera". "You're in luck and might I have the pleasure in seeing you to it and across?"

This was not what Peter was expecting but he asked the man to show him to the crossing and then to see him across. Within himself he was considering the chances of appreciating such synchronicity occurring under different circumstances and asking himself whether or not he would have been aware of the crossing had he been alone with Max. He speculated and thought that maybe he would but he was incredibly grateful.

Up to the crossing, which was literally beside the garage, Max led the progression. Peter was in his wheelchair and the unknown, but helpful, individual walked on the roadside edge of the wheelchair. He pressed the button below the lights and they awaited a response. The oncoming traffic came to a halt, allowing the berated pedestrians to cross. Having successfully traversed the road Peter contemplated the return – back to the bridge (on the other side of the road) and being aware of the intervening distance from his memory, he did not feel that his association with Max could produce a successful progression. He asked if his recent acquaintance would be willing to help him as far as the supermarket, feeling that from there on would be within the capabilities of both himself and the dog.

The aforementioned individual replied that he would be delighted and they duly set off. Before long, what Peter had been aware of, came to pass. The pavement narrowed, leaving an awareness that similar incumbents (in wheelchairs) should be really doing the opposite of what Peter was doing and having crossed at the related crossing, go down the same pavement which he had just come up, arriving back at the Treacy crossing, find themselves effectually barred from association around the town. It was a long way back and no-where to go. A solution was offered; Peters' acquaintance from outside L and M motors suggested leaving the narrowing pavement and braving a path along the edge of the N11. It would allow them a route for getting where it was that was required. He would take the side further into the road and with his stature could expect oncoming cars to take note of his presence and drive accordingly. Accepting the proposal, Peter directed Max to a position on the inside of the three of them and they duly set off. Not being able to actually see the oncoming traffic was at this stage, an advantage for Peter. But he was able to hear both cars and Lorries as they understood and indeed tolerated the trio's intrusion onto the road.

After some distance the pavement had resumed its appropriate width and with an obvious sense of relief the trio returned to the appropriate pavement.

They had passed a building with the name Minch Norton displayed and before long they were rounding the corner as owned by the supermarket. It was here that Peters' acquaintance was to leave them and it was with extreme thanks that Peter bid his new associate farewell. He and Max now considered the way ahead; here they were at a pedestrian crossing, the pavement was cut away (allowing wheelchairs to leave the pavement and be driven down onto the roadway), there were lights in existence to show cars/pedestrians whom it was that would have right of way at a particular moment.

But it was with slight amusement that Peter conceded that a problem now existed. His memory took him back to a conversation amongst his friends, concerning the same pedestrian crossing and a revelation which may have been made by someone in the know. The supermarket, at the time of construction, may have been allowed to build out onto the same corner if they would have been prepared to put in place a pedestrian crossing complete with lights. The crossing was built and the lights (it was reported) caused a disturbance against the flow of traffic proceeding up the N11. The lights were switched off and had not been actively employed since, given that it was suggested that lights would be built in situ. But no disclaimer was made that they should in fact work. Que-sera- sera, whatever will be will be.

Peter was faced with a conundrum; a pedestrian crossing but with no active lights engaged on the same and therefore no audible signal telling him of the appropriateness to cross. Again he was going to have to take his life in his hands and truly depending on Max, instigate a crossing. Dimly he made out the structure of the relevant redundant pedestrian crossing posts; there was no button to press in order to engage them, but with considerably reduced traffic effecting a turn onto the same road (Barrack Street) he was able to cross – showing his dog obviously leading a wheelchair across the road. Success having been achieved he followed the course of the N11, round The Bailey and back down towards the bridge.

Coming to what he knew to be the bottom of Slaney Street, he was presented with a fresh plethora of possibilities. He could either go up Slaney Street, in order to come down Castle Hill, to his prescribed destination or carry on along the N11 until it gave way onto Slaney Place, which in turn would lead him to the castle. Decisions, decisions, decisions, it was always a question and never apparently having an answer.

He knew all of the last few minutes to have been so unnecessary; had it been a weekday Eamon would have been in place, seen him securely across the road and they would have been in this position without the added formality of having to go all the way up the road as far as the L and M Motors. Still, he thought, let's deal with it as we find it. Peter was a realist and forced himself to evaluate the life which had been dealt to him.

He felt himself to be bright and now with Max and his chair he might be considered to have all the redeeming qualities which an actively accomplished and fully participating member of the human race would be capable of demonstrating to the world at large. With his mind-set he was conceding to Keith, who had held the apparently ludicrous opinion that all of this may have been brought into existence for a particular end to be achieved. He could appreciate himself as being a champion for all fellow sufferers of similar conditions to himself and with his intellect and progression; the way ahead was made up of a road which if not leading directly uphill, could be understood to now be levelling out and resorting to a level where victory of progression was within his grasp. He was giving himself a value.

Slaney Street was a street which had always perturbed him, as he knew that at the bottom of it and running directly parallel to the N11 was an area called Mary Street. This held such businesses as Kenny's For Bikes and was it now to be seen as a misnomer, because to a very limited understanding was it to be considered as a street or a square? He pondered on this and knew that the relevant electoral rolls gave out that Mary Street was now surplus to recognised existence. The name had been superseded and Mary Street had now become a part (albeit at right angles to) the appreciated and recognised Slaney Street. Why? Well the Railway had brought about the demise of one Mary Street, in its original manner of running from below Slaney Street up to the present day ascribed Barrack Street, it was seen as an appropriate and recognisable street. But in 1862 the railway had arrived in Enniscorthy and it was designated a very uncertain route into or around Enniscorthy, which was a town centred on a hill moving away from its castle. It was decided to tunnel through the town, allowing the tracks to join from its route into the town from Gorey and the north to a continuous track out towards New Ross and Wexford. This intrusion into the town was going to quite effectually cut Mary Street in half and so what was left was a vastly reduced appreciation of the once inglorious street which had gone by the name of Mary Street and to all appreciation what was left was an apparent square still holding the name.

He decided that his concern was for nothing and that therefore he really ought to continue on his prescribed journey, so with Max leading, in a very fixated and determined fashion the duo entered Slaney Place. So be it if the surface of the prescribed pavement was of an alternating level – it was ideal for pedestrians and he was only in a wheelchair and he knew of no town councillor who was demonstrating the slightest concern for his present predicament, so deal with it. He moved on.

Arriving at the southern end of Slaney Place, he paused outside of The Castle Bar. He knew that he was within accomplishment of his prescribed itinerary, the castle was now within sight (for a normal person) and all that was now required was a 50 meter progression up to the castle gates. But he now conceded that there might perhaps be a possible problem. The route was clear; he aware of it, but it was all to be achieved on a different dimension. The way led up and it was a particularly steep ascent.

He recalled a time when he had attempted this on a motorised bike; a push bike fitted with an engine. Sometime before he had been given a bike of this sort by a friend who had got it for his daughter, but it had now been expended and available for whatever or whoever would take it on. It came from a manufacturer called Fitzgerald and was a decidedly functional and economic unit. A Mountain Bike complete with assisting engine. If the engine was not to be required then it could be disengaged and resume life as a bicycle. On certain ascents or particular journeys, where the engine could be of assistance to the rider, the same bike was of inestimable benefit. However on an occasion where Peter had found himself at the bottom of Castle Hill and having an intention to ascend, the grade of the hill had very nearly proved one of insurmountability. But with dexterity and persistence the expected ascend had been achieved, speaking volumes for the power of the bike (and God bless Fitzgerald).

He considered the wheelchair and appreciating its power source of an electric battery, thought that maybe the gradient of the street might just prove the better of the expended same source of power. Then he thought of the photo opportunity; a man complete with guide dog unable to ascend Castle Hill, it might just prove ideal. Papers and sources of media content were crying out for such instances. Instead he withdrew within himself and settled on achieving his prescribed destination. They faced Castle Hill and with The Castle Bar on the right hand side, started the ascent. He could detect the whine of the electrical accoutrements propelling the chair forward. He accepted, without actually looking, that Max was accompanying him at the side of the wheelchair, but his head was intently turned towards the intended proceedings. The climb began. In a not too obvious fashion, the road meandered towards the left; a straight forward progression with an ample pavement.

17. The Castle

To his relief/surprise he attained the castle gates and appreciated that the expended power from the wheelchair had been something for which he hadn't actually planned. But something lay ahead of him which he had not planned for either. They progressed towards the castle door, it revealed being firmly closed. Perhaps he had made a mistake; there was no great wind apparent to reveal a cause or need to keep the door closed. He directed Max to adopt a sitting position to his right-hand side whilst he deliberated. He had detected no signs revealing opening hours so imagined numerous forms of distress to have occurred within the premises resulting in the closure of the same door.

As he contemplated the immediate predicament he was suddenly aware of an individual approaching his position from the same gates which he had just come through (it was the only entrance to the castle). The person came up and in a broad southern drawl (American) enquired as to Peter holding the position that he was. Peter explained his confusion as to the door being closed and asserted his predicament as to *obvious* health concerns which he was entertaining. The American countered by declaring that the hotel had told him that the castle was not opening until 12.30 (it was now just after 10.30) but that he had thought that with his schedule for the day fully made up, he would see if the castle was open, just with no guides being available until 12.30. Peter laughed and told him that this was Ireland, that it was the year it was and with society behaving as it did, it was not going to be clever to leave a castle unattended overnight with people able to have access to untold valuable and irreplaceable historical icons.

Peter turned from the door and immediately became aware of a dark shape, out between him and whatever was surrounding the castle environs. He moved onto the grass and enquired of his new associate the relevance of the same. "Well back in the hotel they told us that in the grounds of the castle we would see the anchor of the Pomona. Do you know what that is?" Peter, in an attempt to sound knowledgeable whilst at the same time endeavouring to maintain some sort of comprehension, expressed surprise. "The Pomona was one of the ship wrecks off the Irish coast to contribute to one of the largest loss of life in a maritime accident. In 1859 the Pomona had sunk with a loss of life of nearly 400. But this I don't understand; I can feel that this is an anchor", he was moving his hands over the available tenure and shaking his head in disbelief. "You say that this is the anchor off the Pomona, I can feel that it is indeed an anchor and a dated one at that but my understanding is that down in a place called Kilmore Quay – in a memorial garden, there is something giving itself out as being the anchor of the same Pomona. I can feel that this particular anchor has a wooden cross spar at the top and the one down in Kilmore Quay is entirely metal. 'Something smells in Denmark', I know from my study that the Pomona was a two anchored ship, so we could assume that there is one in each place, but this one is so utterly different to my memory of the one down in Kilmore Quay that they could be off different ships. If this gets out it may make me Mr. Popular for the South-East. An anchor in Enniscorthy and an anchor in Kilmore Quay, both claiming for whatever reason to be off the one ship, allowing one party to remember and the other party to gain knowledge, I don't think so. From my memory, even the spades at the base of each anchor are entirely different. Someone may have to explain but with the limitation of opening hours" he said with contempt, "the staff may just be inside now sorting out this confusion".

The American didn't quite know what he was talking about and in his embarrassment and bewilderment sulked away out of the castle grounds, leaving Peter to turn his wheelchair away from the anchor and in turn himself, leave the castle domain.

The route immediately after leaving the castle was now so much less of a strain on the resources of the wheelchair given that he was now going downhill. Together, he and Max arrived outside of The Castle Bar and here Peter had to think. The ridiculous distance involved in returning the way he had initially arrived at where he was, from the hotel and the immediacy of a route which he knew that with assistance he could now achieve. With diminishing sight he looked in the direction of the bridge and pondered. He thought of the ridiculous outcome of his most recent endeavours and how he had messed up on not knowing the opening hours for the castle. He had assumed that he would have known the opening hours, but no and it was not appropriate to look anywhere else to cast blame, it was his alone and now, could he understand having gained anything from his bungled wheelchair saunter around Enniscorthy?

He had come to concede that in all reality society was always available to make its own excuses and to always justify its stance as regards a given position which it was going to hold. People were fickle and always, apparently wanting to self-justify. But just when things appeared to be at their worst – a surprise, a person or an event would come into existence who would serve to remedy, or rectify whatever situation was appearing to hold a non-solution. He gazed towards the bridge and whether as a result of his present thought pattern or whatever, he deduced a darkened form. He performed his (by now) usual double take and forced his concentration to make sense of what he perceived; a shape, a person (definitely), some source of possible assistance – ya!

He was looking towards the bridge and this shape was standing just outside of what he knew was The Credit Union. Dog and wheelchair moved towards the shape and as he drew closer Peter suddenly came to realise that what he had been looking at had now gained the predilection of a Garda.

The Garda was looking away from Peter and down towards the bridge. He was in fact observing some young lads engaged in fishing. He hadn't noticed Peter and his descent down the hill. So as Peter approached him from the castle side of where he was standing, it was with an apparent shock that Peter now revealed himself. Knowing that he had got the attention of a Garda Sciochana, Peter ventured to enquire as to the possibility of the Garda being of assistance to him. He was asked of what benefit the Guard could be and seeing the dog, was slightly apprehensive of the assistance which he might be in a position to offer. However the body language of the same Garda (unseen by Peter) spoke volumes and made it perfectly obvious that required assistance would be available.

Peter merely explained his predicament and boldly enquired as to the possibility of receiving assistance in his aim of making it to the hotel. The Garda was only too delighted to provide the required assistance and even suggested that he would see Peter up as far as the hotel. Gratefully Peter accepted this unasked for help and with nothing more to say, the Garda stepped onto the road running over the bridge and immediately brought the traffic availing of the N11; at that point, to a halt.

Peter directed his wheelchair towards the Garda in order to take advantage of the situation. Max, in perfect obedience, attained a role of complete subservience and walked along at the side. They crossed the N11 just before the western end of the upper bridge and the three proceeded up towards the Treacy pedestrian crossing.

Peter sought to intrude into the pervading silence which had come to exist between himself and the Garda, "Not the usual employment for a guard positioned around the bridge, eh?" "Seeking only to help,

Sir" had been the reply. Where the pavement attained an appropriate width for the passage of one wheelchair alone, the garda had availed of the roadway in order to move closer to the hotel. The oncoming traffic, coming up the road towards Oulart, took the expected action and either moved out into the road in order to pass the guard or else came to a halt until the same guard had incited a situation allowing them to pass.

In this way they approached the intended pedestrian crossing and with obvious indifference the garda turned to leave. Peter, however, regaled the same official by expressing his thanks and suggesting that had he received such assistance from representatives who were in a position to ensure that people facing his predicament, were facilitated with the required support which might be their wont to expect, Enniscorthy could have become a form of haven for wheelchair users. The Garda responded with just one word "money". He turned and left.

Peter and Max had been left on the Treacy side of the crossing and so it was relatively easy to gain the attention of the reception clerk, in order to avail of the disabled entrance to the hotel. They entered and moving along the prescribed route, over towards the bar, Peter took his mobile from where it was secured on the chair and phoned Dave. He asked to be picked up and concluded that his being so would then mark an end to his Enniscorthy adventure.

18. Brittas Bay

Returning to his home and understanding the success (or not) of his recent itinerary, Peter reflected on his achievements to date. With Keith in America, busy finding out the suitability for him to move to America and exist in a wheelchair, whilst he had remained back home in Ireland; learning of different stories relating to areas close to his home. He knew that scenic appreciation was not within his grasp but the spoken word disclosed to him by locals of a related area, were of a value which he could retain. He had gained an insight into the village of Kilmuckridge and he had gained awareness from people whom he would otherwise not have met. He had elected to renew his acquaintance, once more, with Enniscorthy; a town which he thought he had known but by having sought to acquaint himself with unfamiliarity's, he had come to the understanding that unfamiliarity breeds contempt and surprise awaits the unwary.

He now sought to move his point of interest further afield and allow himself an increased area of concern; he had appreciated that Brittas Bay might well be an area which, apart from its reputation for being a wonderful holiday destination, might hold significance for him, having remembered that, as a family, they had holidayed there in the past.

He found himself investigating and making plans accordingly. He didn't think that the sea would be closed (like the castle) or that his being there was going to be dependent on people, on tides, or whatever. He arranged for Dave to drive him up to the beach and whilst leaving him there, be in a position to pick him up later. Dave had concerns in the area to contend with, whilst Peter would be satisfying his curiosity pertinent to the beach.

As regards other concerns which could be construed to be available for Peter; Dad was completely involved with work and therefore might be understood to not have time to expend on his son. Helen (his mother) was engaged with employment in the library and could not allow herself appropriate time in order to make the visit a joint adventure. Tim was felt to be too far outside the immediate sense of intimacy which Peter felt that he could cope with and his best friend Keith was still in America; expected back shortly. He had closed down his association with people to one of involvement with just these four people and his own personae wouldn't allow him to expand this association. He was feeling insecure and vulnerable, he wanted time alone.

The weeks had gone by with Peter just withdrawing into himself. He felt his inadequacies and as a consequence of his not being able to blame anyone else for his predicament, the hole which he was creating was just getting bigger. His voice was now all but finished; his balance was now dependent on the sides of the wheelchair holding him (supporting his imagined posture), but the one redeeming asset which he now still retained, to some extent, was his eyesight. It had diminished in the standard being made available to him but he knew that he was still able to distinguish shape, size and colour. Never mind detail, a bonus which he found that given the other three characteristics being in place was tolerable to be without. But his appreciated value as a living, breathing, mobile entity was gone. He felt valueless. He was distancing himself from everyone. With hesitancy, the fab four (or rather three, because Keith was still in America) would endeavour to approach him, but the self-pitying shape (which was what he had allowed himself to become) was becoming intolerant to all but the most pressing and immediate concerns. He knew and indeed recognised how anti-social he was appearing but the self-pitying was bigger than his need to share.

What had he to share? If indeed he had anything, who was going to want it?

His mind still retained his personality and he would allow his mind to do a great deal of thinking. The thoughts may have been misguided or even incorrect, but they were his thoughts and they contributed to the personality which he was becoming. He was hurting those people who most cared for him and he knew it. But what lay ahead for him? He was forced to consider his own mortality, a boy of nineteen and with damn all prospects. "This is it. This is as far as I go. There is nothing else, oh dear".

But wait. It was under these self-same instances, these very thoughts that miracles were expected to reveal themselves. A person sank to their very depths, depths with no sign of improvement, no light at the end of the tunnel, nothing to permit the existence of hope and then with all else failing; an event, a cure, a wondrous occurrence. Well that was the way it worked in fiction. It was always the hero always coming out, at the end, cured, healed and perfect. It made for nice print but why not move it over into reality? Was Now so big, so incomprehensible that there was no room for anything other than comprehended happenings occurring?

To get a result, was it always necessary to mentally cajole, to push, to seek to make bargains, to build an imagined world where all was right, everything was perfect and intolerance would not be allowed? To be answerable to no-one and ultimately concede that as the flow of thought was all one way, no response was ever going to be required.

What did all this mean and where was it leading? Bring it down to basics. Was the resultant flow of expended energy simply going to be lost somewhere? Was it going to rest and be lost in the space between his ears? With thoughts like these, Peter, alone against the world (his world) was looking to nothing, for nothing, seeing nothing to enable him to need to pick himself up, brush himself off and renew association with a world which he recognised as cold, indifferent and most of all uncaring.

Possession, being reputedly, nine tenths of the law, allowed him to go that extra mile. He could claim complete possession of his entire deteriorating body and sod the begrudgers. He saw himself as a deteriorating entity, one of limited value – he had no value (to himself). Within his mind he could only see a refugee without a homeland. No singular possession to make a claim of an ability to share. He was, in all truth, existing and deteriorating simply because he was missing the capability to share. He was thinking as a freshly diagnosed stoic, an incumbent recently diagnosed with M.S... He had that other part but he was failing to see it. If he could extend his self-centeredness to include a wider appreciation than the mind-set which his mentality was allowing him and see that strength co-existed everywhere, life was going to include a greater degree of accomplishment than he might be prepared to admit.

For now his thoughts turned towards Brittas Bay and whatever experiences were awaiting his ability to absorb and learn from. All things pertaining to the journey had been discussed with Dave and arrangements were in place. The day selected had proved to be one of glorious temperatures and sunshine. Blue skies and extended visibility ensured that having left the N.11 at Jack Whites (a restaurant), to avail of a route to Brittas Bay, the first entry to the beach area being The Southern Car Park, was fully congested with holiday makers or day trippers, so Dave proposed The North Car Park. It was here that Dave deposited Peter along with Max. Dave had been reluctant to merely leave Peter in such an obviously vibrant location, but Peter had allowed him to know that with his shadow and ever-willing aide (accomplice) Max, he need have no concern and that the bond which now was in place between them was sufficient to ensure a degree of accomplishment in their coming endeavours.

The wheelchair was unloaded, with Peter securely in place and as he moved the forward control, in order to propel the chair in a direction which would take him towards the beach, Max fell in, in his usual spot to the front and the right of the wheelchair. They left Dave, with a slightly concerned air about his usual flamboyant nature and following a tarmacked walkway made their way down onto the beach.

Peter was seeing the sea to his front, with sand to his left and right and detecting movement all around. He could come to realise that the beach was well attended by the overthrows of somewhere like Dublin. As he brought the ensemble of the three of them (dog, chair and himself) down towards the sea front, the swath of beachgoers parted, allowing him easy access in his endeavours to attain the water's edge. He failed to comprehend that perhaps they were displaying a wish to disassociate themselves with having to be of assistance to an invalid who could bring about a ruination of their day being spent with no concerns of such a nature.

Max, whilst being ever attendant, was displaying a wish to involve himself in more. He wished to play. He continually would turn his head towards the wheelchair, hoping for a release direction which would effectively remove him from responsibility for the chair and permit him to break away and partake in play time, yards from them now, within the sea.

Peter, understood from the appropriate noises coming to him from the beach area, that all was conducive of a normal day where people would avail of the distractions of the seaside in order to distance themselves from the resulting mediocrity of a day spent employed at industry, commerce or whatever.

He elected to involve himself in participation by thinking of himself as just one more of a forgotten crowd partaking of inclusion within the beach area. Concerned that perhaps the sand would not bear the weight of his chair, he gingerly edged his way onto the beach. Satisfied that the surface tension was sufficient to support him and chair, he proceeded with a heightened sense of security. Nearing the water's edge, he allowed Max the freedom for which he was searching.

Max, in his gratitude at being released, turned his body towards the chair and in appreciation stretched out his head. He carefully, extending his head, moved his muzzle over Peters' hand and with much enthusiasm gave Peter a heartfelt compassionate lick; his tongue leaving a damp patch on the back of Peter's right hand. Max broke away and raced into the sea, allowing Peter a silence which he was unaccustomed to – always having the dog in his arc of responsibility. He maintained a dutiful watch (given his available eyesight) on the dog, who was frolicking freely just within his depth.

The dog raced back and forward, in front of him and Peter spent the time in contemplation. He considered how after all the time since his diagnoses; the physical attributes which he now displayed had never progressed to the extent of ever getting in any way what could be described as getting better or showing improvement.

Peter knew that he could command a hall of people, make them aware of the difficulties of his situation and beg them to consider that his was the worst case of M.S. in existence, no-one had more and no-one had worse, let's all feel sorry for Peter. Aw, poor me!

His mind was far removed from any physical plane of existence and without his perception an individual had past close in to where Max was busy displaying self-centeredness himself. Max had no concern or even knowledge of this persons' presence and continued at his play, aware that Peter was going to give him undivided attention. The person swam past.

Minutes rolled by, each individual lost in their own concern; Peter knowing how cruel that the world could be and Max rushing about, yards into the water, behaving as if he were busy inventing every game in the world and demonstrating the moves to an extremely interested congregation. The person swam back, behind Max and suddenly ceasing in his forward motion from propulsion as a result of breaststroke, sank beneath the surface. Max continued and Peter, only half remembering the man having even been there at all, continued with his self-pitying.

Suddenly, in response to Max and his splashing about, throwing the surface of the water into some form of disarray, the man's hand broke the surface and in an uncontrolled fashion his shoulders and torso followed. They fell immediately back into the water. No sound came from the man and if it were not for the lack of forward movement, joking might have understood to have been occurring. He broke the surface again and this time Peter felt, without knowing why, he was looking at a distraught face as the body inhaled a quantity of air. Peter locked his attention on the disappearing man and understood that with all his presented attributes, he could do nothing. He was failing in his self-centredness to appreciate that a degree of eyesight and physicality was returning to him.   Max, appreciating the fact that Peter was no longer focused on him turned, in order to see this new point of interest. He spied the third rise to the surface of the now unstruggling and indeed unconscious 'man of significance'.

Understanding that this was an individual who was requiring assistance, Max turned. His back to the beach, he earnestly looked around and seeing where it was that Peter had directed his attention, throwing his body against the waves struck out for the area. He came to the related area and with no sign of anyone, knew that the object of his concern must be beneath the surface.   He dived, an unaccustomed environment and one not going to allow him immediacy of movement, however in the distance (through the murky water) he spied his target.   Paddling desperately through an unaccustomed media of progression he came to the inert man. Eagerly grabbing the extended arm, he struck out for the surface. Behind him, the body had fallen into place, following the extended arm; they all broke the surface together. Max changed his grip, from the arm of his subject; he now moved his grip to one of getting hold of the man's hair. Being aware of the direction of the shore, he made for it, knowing that whatever he now had in his mouth needed the attention of those whom he knew awaited them.

People avoiding the wheelchair along the edge of the water, now came having seen and understood the gravity of what had just transpired. As the dog brought the unconscious body in to the beach, people clamoured around and very quickly the entire picture changed.

"It's Henry" and people only stood in mute silence as the weight of the moment hit them.

Henry was immediately recognisable from his world accepted profile. Instantly appreciated to be the most significant and lauded man in the realms of his chosen niche. He was a man whom the world could call their own. Attractive in a mature sense and fabulously wealthy, he had never been known to want for anything and now, here he was lying unconscious on a beach, here in Ireland.

After the shock and immediacy of the moment had passed, people collected themselves and an air of normality reigned. Someone, with a mobile suggested calling for an ambulance and when this proposal was adopted the interminable wait held heavy with them all. Maternal matrons moved in, attempting to take charge, coveting their God given prize which they felt had come about through some divine incident. One or two of 'the boys' took over; ever eager to boost themselves and feeling that an opportunity was presenting itself for a degree of image building. Finally the Lifeguards took over and started to direct everyone.

The Ambulance arrived and it careered onto the beach and personal leapt out. All over confusion reigned again and everyone was feeling that they might have an input into saving Henrys' life.

All interest in Max had dissipated and with no-one to provide a source for his ever available curiosity, he had returned, back to the sea. Frolicking may just be so much more fun, anyway. He passed through the crowds, now assembled to stare in assumed amazement at this source of immediate gossip. He tore across the sand and with a convincing splash re-achieved his sought for destination; The Sea.

He remembered his responsibilities and looking around for Peter, amidst the confusion, splashed up to him. Satisfied that things were as they should be, he turned and raced off into the surf. What wasn't known was that he would never come back again, well not without what happened next, occurring first.

Splashing ensuing, watching occurring and the status quo being attained; all appeared right with the world and living was seen to be continuing. Suddenly and with no warning Max (amidst mid splash) froze. His body attained a form of paralyses, locking his various extensions in a fixed and unnatural manner. He whined throughout the unfamiliarity of the occurrence and falling back into the water achieved a comatose appearance.

Very quickly, Peter had perceived what had occurred and through instinct, had made a move to leave the chair. Six months (and the rest) had not allowed him to understand that movement from him was not on. Transfixed he came to the realisation of what he couldn't do. He was unable to rush into the water in order to affect a rescue. Immediately thoughts rushed through his mind; how ridiculous the situation was, having just brought about a rescue of another individual, Max was now in need of assistance himself, that the only person aware of the enfolding situation (himself) was completely unable to render aid in any practical sense. He couldn't even shout to other people; in order to make them aware of their required physical participation. His eyes were making out the entire events and without being aware of it, his perception had gained clarity. For another individual he was now experiencing fear. Terror had taken a hold of him; he knew in that moment that he was simply a pair of eyes.

Forcing him to behave in a fashion dictated by his imagined limitations Peter closed his mind down and became aware of his rigid left small finger. He was forcing his attention onto the digit when suddenly it started to rise. It had not moved for weeks and the movement had an all entrancing, surreal effect on Peter and his mental awareness. He was moving a finger.

Once again, centred only on himself, he speculated on what else was possible. He regarded his frozen centre finger, again on his left hand. Forcing his mind on the sole digit – it too moved. In wonderment, Peter worked through-out his body, demanding without contradiction, the movement of related areas. He found himself suggesting a quiver (or shake) to come from his right leg, it responded. Through-out his body, parts suddenly came to life and all because Peter was requiring it to be so. He would not see another reason for this occurring except for his self-centred interest in attaining his original physical wellbeing.

He felt that his posture in the chair had suddenly achieved a new propensity, he was sitting taller, straighter and he was becoming appreciative of feeling the dimensions of the wheelchair. Sensations of which he had been unaware were now beholden to him and still he was accepting this to all be as a result of his own volitions; meaning that after all he was still looking no further than himself.

Splashing from the water in front of him brought his psych back to an appreciation of what was occurring immediately to his front. Instantly he speculated on the impending events which he was now going to endeavour to bring into existence. He fixed his gaze on the dog's body, now a reclining feature floating on the surface of the water, at some distance from him. Staring intently, he rose. The wheelchair fell behind him and for the first time in months Peter stood, unaided by assisting artificial supports, he progressed forward into the water. With the determination of the moment, he fixed his mouth in an unaccustomed grimace and strode on. The water rose above his ankles and still he progressed. His knees were now covered by the level of The Irish Sea and the dog was closer. Step by step (each step an unconscious movement brought back by memory) Peter was moving towards his one true friend. A companion, who by his very unmoving posture was begging by his demeanour for the association of the two of them; he required rescuing. The water level on Peter came to waist height and still he pressed on. Intention decried that yards separated the pair from a reunion which would result in a renewing of association to the benefit of them both. Max needed a rescue and Peter required retaining his present position of well-being.

Peter came up alongside of the now floating, inert body; Max's head was dragging along under the surface of the water and all movement had ceased. The suspension of the water may have been a help in the support of Peters' body but in order to clasp Max he would now have to lift his arms clear of the surface of the water and grasp his friend. Urgency demanded immediacy and Peter staring at his friend raised his arms and threw them forward enclosing the dog.

Altering his stance on the bottom of the sea, Peter turned his body back to the shore. Max was floating, now with his head clear of the water and in unison the pair returned to the beach. People who had been pre-occupied with the Henry situation now came to understand that a different scenario was taking place and one which would command utterly different responses from entirely different people.

An unoccupied wheelchair was observed, by the edge of the sea, the occupant was now observed wadding, coming back in towards the shore. Disgust registered on the demeanour of congregated observers and knowing no better they turned away in disgust. There were however others, who far from putting the existence of the wheelchair alongside this misconceived association of the wadding youth, looked further and saw that the same youth was in the process of now bringing to shore a golden shape of some substance.

"Another body?" " A seal?" "It's just some garbage!" The questions were passed around in an unanswered fashion and concern was extended towards the youth. Was that his wheelchair? Had he really left it in order to simply pick up some garbage? Could he really have the nerve to be using the wheelchair in order to gain some unknown advantage on an otherwise packed beach? All these and more were the tone of the questions emanating from the bemused onlookers and all this time Peter and Max were making their way to the water's edge.

One or two individuals, of a concerning nature, raced into the water to be of whatever assistance may be required. As they approached the duo, they understood that the flotsam being grasped by the youth was in fact a dog; the very dog which had brought about Henry and his presence on their very beach; which they were standing on right at that time. They sensed the gravity of the moment.

They wadded forward and taking Max away from Peter, they all made their way to shore. With the momentary pressure (tension) of the moment gone and no-longer a need to display any supernatural capabilities; Peter was beginning to revert to his previous standard of existence. He fell forward and face down in the water struggled with his own individualism, he got his face above the surface. He spluttered and coughing up a quantity of water found himself unable to stand. He had to accept that the previous minutes, showing his ability to become a living, breathing, fighting entity had all happened simply because of a greater cause. Perhaps his mind had been the inducement for the rescue of Max, but old habits die hard and Peter was still looking only as far as himself in order to explain what had just occurred.

The ambulance was just leaving the beach and people close enough to alert them made them aware that a further issue was just then resulting which may require their attention. The vehicle stopped and a paramedic got out. Enquiries ensued and deliberations were acted on. The same paramedic made his way onto the beach and with an attitude of disbelief urged the youth up to the ambulance.

Peter was not going to leave Max and it was with some interaction that it was agreed that as Max could be considered a guide dog he should accompany Peter in the ambulance. The next thing to do was get Peter to the same vehicle. He was lying on the sand at the edge of the sea and the wheelchair was some distance away. The paramedic was unaware of the situation which had just transpired, so, assuming that Peter had fallen off from the wheelchair, the wheelchair was retrieved from where it lay further along the beach and with some difficulty Peter was returned to it.

All that Peter was interested in was the condition of Max. He was soaking wet and the paramedic, in desperation, returned to the ambulance and getting a colleague came back to Peter with a stretcher. Between the two of them they were capable of taking Peter from his wheelchair, placing him in the stretcher and with someone else carrying Max, they all came back to the ambulance.

Henry appeared to have the right of priority (being the cause of the ambulance being there anyway) and Peter was moved to a very secondary position. Concern was now extended towards Max, who was shivering but having shown a propensity of life that was taking attention off him and (rightly?) back onto Henry. The paramedic administered massage upon the dog (not having suitable alternative remedies) and conceding that the dog may have suffered a heart tremor of some proportion felt that there was little else which he could do.

Henry had regained consciousness and looked with some curiosity at the acquired payload of the ambulance. He enquired as to the reason for him having to share a ride wherever, in such company. The attendant paramedic, in some awe at having Henry in the ambulance and unaware of the entire situation, merely stated that the youth and the dog were also just after having suffered an incident of some proportion, back on the beach. It was thought that it was entirely coincidental that the two incidences had occurred at the same time, on the same beach.

Peter had heard all of these disclosures and sought to bring some finality to the proceedings. He attempted to reveal the actual occurrence of events but found that with the engine noise of the ambulance and his own level of speech, he was unable to do so. There was an obvious air of disassociation between the pair in the back of the ambulance.

Max stood up and moving over to the most convenient reclining position in the vehicle, seeing that it was occupied by Henry, sought whilst still remaining on the floor, to renew acquaintance.

Henry had always loved dogs and having a special place in his heart for Labradors, responded by stroking Max. He caressed the top of his head and gently toyed with his two ears. Max complemented the action by sinking into a demeanour of subservience, contentment and relaxation. They continued on their journey to Loughlinstown Hospital and it was there, whilst both paramedics went into the hospital in order to determine suitable space that conversation between Peter and Henry could finally take place.

"I see you like Max", enquired Peter and Henry replied in the affirmative. "He appears an incredible well behaved dog". "He's a guide dog", responded Peter. "A guide dog, but for whom?" came the response from Henry. "He's a guide dog for me". "And under what criteria do you qualify for a guide dog?" came Henry's immediate retort, not appreciating that Peter would have a condition meriting the use of a guide dog. "On this bunk, here in this ambulance, I may appear to have nothing wrong with me, but rotate me to a standing position and all might be revealed. You see I have Multiple Sclerosis and Max is a very welcome addition for my condition. Actually it was him who rescued you". This came as a shock to Henry who had no idea how he had got to his present position. "I don't remember. The last thing of which I am aware is swimming at a beach, just south of Dublin, In fact how I came to be here, I have no idea". "You were swimming at Brittas Bay, just opposite me when I think you had a stroke or something. Max saw your condition and he saved you, he returned to the water after making sure that there were people looking after you and as soon as he got into the water, the same thing happened to him".

"Are you telling me that I owe my life to this dog", it was at this juncture that the paramedics arrived back and they immediately took Henry and placing him on a trolley, they wheeled him into the hospital. Peter was very much a secondary concern and with his self-imposed isolation of the last six months, he had been unaware of whom Henry had been. They never saw each other after this and Peter was duly discharged from Loughlinstown Hospital later that day. He was stumped, his wheelchair was still down at Brittas Bay and his mobile had been secured to it, he had no immediate means of getting in contact with Dave.

Dave meanwhile had found out about the happenings at Brittas Bay and having being there had accepted recovery of the same wheelchair, complete with mobile etc. He had learnt that the participants in the day's activities had been taken to Loughlinstown Hospital and had gone there himself in order to acquaint himself with the state of play.

Upon Peter being discharged from the hospital, contact was made between himself and Dave, and they were able to get back home with a range of adventures to reveal. But Peter now had some serious issues to explain, if only to himself. He thought long and hard and with no conclusions. Nothing was presenting itself as having been the cause, or even the effect, of whatever he had been through. He recognised the fact that Max had been the concern which had brought the occurrence into being. He knew that at some point he had lost all of his disability and at the point in time of this happening, he could have competed with the world's best; competed and won. He knew that he loved Max and there was a bond between them that passed all understanding. For Max, he would have laid down his life, but was all of this sufficient to bring into existence this lapse of attained vulnerability, this contrite subjection, this physical susceptibility which he had experienced. He couldn't see and then he had looked with other eyes; he stopped seeing the subjective and turned it around so that the objective was what concerned him. He stepped away and considered the entire picture from another perspective. No more would he permit himself to consider "I" or "me", now there were other people and issues to contend with. The world was bigger and consisted of fewer people (a conundrum!) each with their own story, their own slant on life and with their own answers to selected problems. If he should bring himself to see that, at the end of it all, we are all one, sharing a common goal, a hoped for ending, without differentiation, then suddenly all can be achieved and utopia could be attained. Stop all this selfish self-centredness and self-interest, MOVE ON!

He was finding himself to be a new person; a completer and more fulfilled individual; a happier and more content being. He had not regained his full faculties which he had known before, but now with a fuller understanding for his own circumstances, he could tolerate a great many more things than he had been prepared to condone before.

As he remained at home waiting for Keith, he was able to see himself being a more accepting person. He knew that with certain parameters in place, things had a propensity for change. He hadn't yet come to know the complete unselfishness required to break a form of permanency to any outcome. Still he was preserving that ethos which told him that it was sufficient to look no further than himself. He was allowing a pattern of thought which told him that all things were being brought into place simply (or only) through the power of the mind.

He was becoming more outward looking and found himself willing to share more of a condition which he had come to recognise as simply himself. In the evenings Peter would allow himself to fraternise with the remainder of his family and it was on just such an occasion that he found his life taking another turn.

19. Late-Late Show

It was a Friday evening shortly after his adventure pertinent to Brittas Bay. Helen had suggested an evening spent in front of 'The Box'. She had understood that Peter appeared to have gone through a form of epiphany in relations to his approach with other people. This was a picture which she wished to encourage and so they were all assembled in the sitting room – adjacent to Peter's space behind the recently constructed wall. The wheelchair was in a significant position and everyone was gathered with apparent enthusiasm. The News had just ended and a program called The Late-Late Show was about to start.

For an unknown reason silence had befallen the room and intense interest was being shown towards the regarded screen. Ryan Tubridy came onto the screen and made the following announcement; "It is with particular enthusiasm that we bring the following to your attention. The entire show may very well be given to this one particular topic. It is of significant interest to a large proportion of the Irish population both as regards sufferers as well as carers. But to introduce this topic I am going to introduce you to an individual who bears no need for introduction and will be extremely well known to you. Known to you all and recognised simply by one name, Ladies and Gentlemen, I give you Henry"

A figure appeared at the back of the studio and came forward. Dressed in clothes revealing casual acceptance for the moment, he came and sat down where Tubridy had directed him. Everyone was left with the question of what was going to transpire, as they had all attended the show, that evening, expecting a usual show of chat, singing and demonstration. This was unexpected, but was it just another quirk or twist coming from The Late-Late Show.

Drawing himself up to appear bigger than his six foot four, Henry took over the screen and told the audience that he faced a particular problem. He had recently had an experience which may be of interest to the watching masses. He told how he had been swimming at a beach, south of Dublin; called Brittas Bay. Whilst pursuing this activity he had had a heart attack. His life could be seen to have been coming to an end but suddenly he was aware that he was in an ambulance, heading back to Dublin. He found that he had had to share the ambulance with an unusual pair; a youth and a dog. The apparent ignominy of the company and also that he had no full understanding of how he had got to where he was allowed Henry to be slightly perplexed by the activity. The dog had approached him and in some sort of bewilderment he had endeared himself to the dog. The youth sitting opposite to him had initially appeared mute, having showed signs of wanting to say something but then deciding to leave words unspoken. It had only been when they had got to the hospital that a chance occurred when he could express himself. He went on to explain that the dog had in fact been responsible for saving Henry (who apparently had had a heart attack).

All of this was happening on the big screen. Whilst this was being revealed Peter was saying nothing. He recognised Henry as being the subject in the ambulance and he would every so often throw his eyes up to the ceiling. After his misadventures in Brittas Bay he had sworn Dave to secrecy, fearing that Max would have been taken off him.

Henry continued and went on to say that he had; as a result of revelations made in the back of the ambulance, made investigations as to the identity of the pair, but had come up with nothing. As a direct result of his position Henry had usurped the evening's presentation of The Late-Late Show and was going to use it for several purposes. First of all, he was seeking to know of the identity of the reluctant heroes and then he was going to further the cause of Multiple Sclerosis which the youth had said that he was afflicted with.

Helen expostulated and was beside herself. "Peter, darling, you were down in Brittas Bay. You have M.S., maybe it's you he's talking about". She said all this in jest, knowing that after his visit Peter had said nothing and therefore with nothing to say, nothing could have happened.

"Yeah, it's me alright. Max must have saved him and never told me about it". Peter was beginning to understand the seriousness of the situation. The future of the pairing of himself and Max was suddenly going to be brought into the light; he knew that he had not lied about anything that had occurred at Brittas Bay but by understanding simple family association he knew that he should have said something. He wasn't overawed by the appearance of Henry; indeed he was just a person in an ambulance who had stroked his dog. But what Henry had done as regards taking over The Late-Late Show brought a line of questioning into Peters' mind.

Dad was sitting, saying nothing but watching Peter and his reaction to disclosures coming from the box. He had been approached by Dave and told of all that had happened down in Brittas Bay, on the day in question. He looked at it in such a way as to understand that nothing could be achieved by reacting in any other way then had been actually done. He knew how important was the pairing of his son with Max and that this should be encouraged. Very carefully and subtly he had kept a closer eye on the two since the Brittas Bay excursion and realising the importance of the pairing had just kept a watching eye. He wished to assist his son in this delicate moment by taking the pressure off, but the fact that a significant show such as The Late-Late was now going to have its entire time given over to disclosures from Henry; it didn't seem to be exactly appropriate to suggest a change of channel.

A joke! "Maybe Max knew who he had rescued and thought it would be better to say nothing". Peter understood half the game that his father was playing and supported his words by adding "and we'd have got a free ride in an ambulance".

But further disclosures were going to come from Henry. Attention was angled towards the TV and he went on to reveal that he had not, at any stage been in a satisfactory position to describe the youth by physical appreciation but, he went on to say that the Labrador had been a golden retriever. Helen, with no real knowledge of dogs pertinent to types, thought that a golden retriever was long haired and that therefore it could not be Max who was under discussion. "Thought it might have been you, Max", she said reaching down to the dog, reclining in a subservient position at Peters feet.

The pressure was now off and watching of the program could continue. Henry had other disclosures to make and Peter had further ceilings to regard. But throughout, Helen appeared satisfied that her knowledge of the dog, in question, would not allow Max in any way to be involved. But still she wondered and with the wondering came unanswered questions. She watched the show with an interest which came from the hoped for disclosures relating to Multiple Sclerosis.

The programme continued with instances being revealed by Henry of the magnitude of the M.S. situation occurring in the world (and pertinent to Ireland). His team of researchers had visited areas around the country contaminated by this affliction and had interviewed incumbents with the condition. The family watched in amazement and saying nothing, they remained transfixed by revelations disclosed. It was revealed the range of symptoms amenable to this particular plight and although Peter could relate to the vast majority of them; such things as lack of mental focus or agility had not been a symptom experienced by him.

Songs were included in the show with lyrics which appeared to sum up the entire situation pertaining to individuals so encumbered:

POEM: - *I can hear the wind that's blowing,*

But I can't see the trees it shakes

I'm dependent on my physic

And the memoires of out-takes.

Dad said nothing but with a conciliatory look on his face, he was regarding his son with subtle interest. Knowing the details of the Brittas Bay occurrence and the appreciation of the resultant outcome, he had simply regarded Peter with an interest which said that the outcome would be the outcome. Helen however knew nothing of the Wicklow events and was still accepting Peter to not be the initial cause of, or a contributor to, Henry being in the position in which he was. But something was niggling at her. Dave had said that after Peter had being at Brittas Bay, he had simply picked him up and returned home, but she still wondered.

The show continued and Peter suddenly expostulated that he wished to avail of a course of action which he had (surprisingly!) not planned for. Earlier he had been preparing to get into his bed and he had separated himself from his catheter, his mother had called for him to join them in the sitting room; in order to watch the goggle box and share the evening. As a result of the insisted urgency of the moment, he had forgotten to 'plug himself back in'. He had come into the sitting room along with Max and securing a particular position in the room, had remained in a position of having to hold his urine until he would have returned to his room. But with the disclosures emanating from the TV, excitement had had a bearing upon Peter's physical propensity. He wished to relief himself and this was a particular time (in his mind) when his parents should be introduced to an alternative Peter and one of which (as far as he was aware) the pair of them would have had no inclination.

"I want to go to the toilet", the little room was in a corner. It was beside the door leading to the hall and immediately Dad had moved in order to be of assistance. Peter turning his face in Dad's direction decreed that this assistance was not going to be required. Helen was transfixed and staring at the individual talking, with wide eyes and wonderment stood as though paralysed.

Peter clutched the arms of the chair – it hadn't been known that he could do this. He straightened himself and bracing himself, pushed forward. He rose and with an extremely fixed appearance he shuffled forward. Both of his parents were dumbfounded. His Father, having been told of the apparent goings on in Brittas Bay, had still to evidence a happening of this sort himself. His mother was rooted to the ground (as if she'd seen a ghost) and unable to say anything, just remained staring. Max, whilst suddenly no-longer being a centre of attention perceived that the goings-on was away from any concern of his and remained lying down.

Peter shuffled away from the Wheelchair and centring his attention on his legs brought about a rotation upon the carpet of the room. He moved across it and with a fixed expression focused on the toilet door, moved in that direction. Seconds were elapsing and apart from the noise of Peter and his legs, nothing more was heard except for the sound coming from the TV.

Having got to the door, Peter halted and his father (as though waking from a dream) hurried to his side. "Peter, this is truly magnificent. Here, let me open the door for you". He duly opened the door and stood back. Peter shuffled through. Having lost sight of her son, Helen regained a quantity of her composure and moving up to her husband stuttered "Ho Ho Wha Wha........." she could say nothing comprehensible. Her husband, holding her close, could only say, "Unbelievable".

Peter concluded his purpose for having left the room and returned.

His father regarded him with unspoken support and moving over towards him, said with absolute conviction "And what just happened there?" Peter had returned to the wheelchair and had appeared to resume his initial propensity within the same confines. Looking towards his feet, he said as if to no-one "I cannot give a reason for what you have just witnessed". Helen stepping forward and thinking that Trish (back in the library) was never going to accept what Helen had just been a participant to regarding, could only say "And how long have you been able to do this?"

The words coming from Peter were spoken with a level of delivery unrelated to their importance or significance. "It has only happened the once before and I don't understand it. When I went to Brittas-Bay it happened for the first time, but I couldn't tell you. If you had known what had happened, my ownership of Max could have been altered and you may have taken him off me. Whatever else occurs, I won't willingly permit that. Max and I have a bond that is like nothing else. He has become so important to me and I could never see a situation happening where we were separated". He was almost crying and moving his eyes away from his feet, they rested on the dog contentedly asleep over by the right front leg of the wheelchair.

Dad placing his arm around his sons' shoulder said in a lowered voice, "This will never happen. What we have just seen, moves us to think that perhaps you may be experiencing some form of remission with your M.S. but it might have been helpful if you had told us this earlier, but understand that whatever, you will only have our unending support in all that you are doing".

"But I don't understand what is happening. What happened in Wicklow may have just been because there was a need for the event to occur. But what was the cause of what you have just seen"?

Still the TV was continuing the disclosures which were being broadcast for the benefit of the nation. Helen, having her appreciation of the recent events, turned the conversation towards a fuller involvement of participants within the room and said, with a note of triumph within her voice, "We'll have to tell The Late-Late and allow them to know that we have an answer to one of their enquiries".

She turned to the telephone sitting on a small table beside the door and dialled a number. "We have him; the person you're looking for". Her excitement would not allow her to break the conversation down to a more intelligible form of disclosure and she didn't realise that, in fact she was just speaking to a researcher.

The researcher stabilised the conversation by enquiring what was the issue concerning the caller. Helen, in her excitement was momentarily flummoxed and didn't know what she was being asked. She had, naively, imagined that her having got through to The Late-Late Show, she would now be talking to Ryan Tubridy himself. The researcher explained that she was through to the desk pertinent to the show and she enquired as to her reason for the call. Helen, finding her demeanour once again, suddenly started to reconsider her reason for calling and allowed the researcher to appreciate that a request had been made; from the show, as to the identity of a particular person. That person was in her house and she expected Henry (who was doing tonight's show) to be made aware of it. The researcher asked her for her phone number and assured her that the show would be in contact. The call was ended and the silence in the sitting room, back in Wexford, was perplexing.

Dad, who hadn't heard any of call except one side of it, enquired as to the result of the same and Helen answered him, as if still in her professional capacity in the library, by saying that they would get back. Peter was, apart from still regarding the ceiling, behaving in a very non-committed fashion and the revelations which were going to be made, by his mother, on his behalf, were not being taken by him to be anything serious. Max remained in his comatose state of being, beside Peter and his right leg.

The telephone rang and hurriedly Helen turned to pick up the receiver. "Hello and you are very welcome to be a part of The Late-Late Show". Henry was now involving Helen in being a live participant in the proceedings coming from the box. She was aware that in that moment her voice was behaving as a stereo echo, seconds after she spoke a phrase into the receiver her words were being repeated from a square construction within the confines of the room. She knew immediately the purpose of the call and enthusiastically responded by interjecting and stating that she was calling to reveal that she was the mother of the sought for individual who was a sufferer of the M.S. condition.

Henry (already in fact being aware of the identity of the sought for youth but not having told the audience the same information) enquired as to where she was calling from. She replied that she was speaking from County Wexford and that her son, Peter, was with them and had gone to Brittas Bay, at the elected time, in order to experience the location. She didn't know of anything more that had happened but if Henry wished to, he could speak with Peter directly.

Henry was still playing the game of *knowing nothing* and for the purpose of the show was continuing with the subterfuge of innocence. He had wished Helen to reveal her relevance to the presented show, by revealing her association/relationship to Peter. She had done so and what she hadn't known was that Henry having already known of Peter and his actual address was merely playing with her.

After being discharged from the hospital himself; after three days, he had enquired as to the identity of the mysterious duo. He was immediately aware of what he had been through and how close things had come to finality for him. The hospital had allowed him to know that they couldn't reveal the details relating to Peter (concerns of confidentiality) but, on the QT had told him that the dog being investigated would give Henry all the details for which he was searching – but the information couldn't come from the hospital itself.

Henry, knowing that the dog was a guide dog, immediately contacted relevant authorities and was directed to a training establishment, which in fact (or by coincidence) was the very institution where Max had been trained. He had described a golden Labrador and an accompanying youth. It was immediately recognised who he was talking about. Henry, being the person who he was, got the relevant info and retaining sought for details, appreciated making use of such a media outlet as The Late-Late Show for a related issue such as M.S. and an understanding of its global attributes. He had every wish to bring about a revelation to Irish society of the requirement (in Henry's opinion) of the promotion of M.S. concerns. He had found out the scale of this condition pertaining to Irish society and the contempt with which this disease was considered.

He had made contact with Bill and it had been disclosed how the trainer had conceded that Max had been one very fundamental dog and how Bill had recognised that Max was going to be outstanding; in whatever regard for life which he was going to come up against. Henry and Bill formed an attachment that was going to bring them a lot closer.

Henry played it to the extent of revealing his joy at having finally got an insight into gaining appreciation of the pair's location and as far as those watching the show were going to be involved, he could now have his gratitude proceed to the next level.

The show had already shown a clip revealing the training of dogs due to be dispatched for the assistance of M.S. sufferers and showing how an involvement with these canine assistants was going to allow these sufferers to achieve a degree of independence otherwise denied them.

Through-out the filming (of which Bill and his participation were fundamental) Henry had in no way alluded to the suggestion that Bill had recognised the dog that had had dealings with the rescue of him and the filming had merely shown the process involved in the training of suitable dogs. Yes, it was (as intended) a wee bit of a tear-jerker and sympathy was being sought from respective viewers. At the conclusion of the film further disclosures had been made, songs had been sung and interviews had been a part of an ever revealing show dealing with society's acceptance for a curse such as was Multiple-Sclerosis with all its accompanying attributes.

In conclusion, contact had now been established with the inherent cause of the show and Henry wished to finish with establishment of a definite connection between himself and Peter. Having known all along of the contact details for Peter and having received the call from Helen, a delay had been initiated by the producers in establishing contact with Helen/Peter and when the call from the studio had been made, Henry was able to play it to the extent of (from Helen's point of view) knowing nothing pertaining to the existence of Peter.

Claiming (quite rightly) that she was unaware of the happenings occurring at Brittas Bay, on the day in question, Helen had alluded to the possibility of a conversation between Henry and Peter. Enthusiastically Henry was quite in agreement with this proposal and it was with a degree of trepidation that the phone receiver was handed over to Peter. He had been aware of both sides of a very one sided conversation, by having listened to the television and it was with a degree of resignation that he had now achieved the pivotal position of speaking with Henry.

Peter listened, waiting for Henry to reveal an intention to communicate. An introduction was made and a question as to the extent of Peter having the relevant diagnoses of M.S. (it being considered unusual that an incumbent with this condition would be somewhere such as at the water's edge in Brittas Bay). Peter concurred by revealing that he had been completely dependent on both his wheelchair and his dog, he added that he was a work in progress.

Henry concurred that this showed Peter having a propensity for humour and suggested that their conversation in the ambulance had not shown this to be a characteristic which Peter had revealed. Now however the interaction between the two of them could become one of mutual interaction and indeed participation. "May I enquire how long you have had M.S. and the stage you are at now, with it?" Henry, apart from being aware of the answer coming, was all the time seeking to have a live television show produced for the benefit of the viewers.

"It's been a condition which I have had now for over six months and in that time it has been closing down around me and allowing me to simply be a person in a wheelchair, dependent entirely on my dog. Therefore when events, such as what happened at Brittas Bay occurred, I was totally unprepared for it and I have no explanation for it".

"This event happening down at Brittas Bay", interrupted Henry, "apart from my immense gratitude for its occurrence. Has it happened on any other occasion"? "Yes, once"! "When was that"? "Tonight" "I beg your pardon" came Henrys immediate conjecture. "It happened tonight, when I was sitting watching this show and I was taken short but having left my catheter in my room, my father sought to take me to the toilet and I immediately responded by disclosing how, I felt, that this was something which I was going to achieve myself. I didn't understand that the two episodes were going to be conjoined by your appearance"

Henry was stumped and stated that he (directly) didn't feel that he had been responsible. But, he suggested, that it was the outcome of what was going to transpire which may reveal a cause for what had occurred happening.

Immediately Peter came back with the suggestion that Henry might want to play a game of football with him or something. He failed to see any cause or reason for the two incidents. Henry (literally taking back control of the show) told Peter that he wished to see a partnering of the two of them, in order to alleviate the concern of M.S. throughout Ireland, if not the world.

He held the opinion that an issue such as M.S. held such a propensity of fear for all the inhabitants of the country (being aware of it) that he felt appropriating a vehicle of information such as The Late-Late Show had been entirely justified. It was a live show and therefore held no time or opportunity for editing of released material. "You got what you are watching" and "The truth will out". Ryan Tubridy had adopted the responsible stance by permitting Henry to usurp his presentation, for this one night, in order to get this message of immediate concern out to the watching masses. Henry had not given out a message declaring to all that as a result of watching this show a person is going to get all the answers to M.S., but that by taking on board all that had been delivered a viewer was going to be more informed then they would have been with imagined information. He had brought Max to the fore; this dog (who directly) had actually saved his life and in appreciation Henry was showing his gratitude by revealing to all that a use, or a purpose, was existing whereby these canines could be used as an active and real assistant to an individual with such a pressing concern as M.S..

To the viewer's understanding, he had achieved the initial purpose which he had set out to do; he had discovered the identity and location of this elusive pair. Peter had not sought immediate anonymity and disassociation from the event. Rather he had, apart from not realising the significance of Henry, sought to bring into existence a situation whereby the union between himself and Max could be preserved. He had been aware that Max had actually saved Henry and he had always suspected the gratitude felt by Henry for his friend. But this was tempered by his knowing that if the story had got out to his parents; that Max had had a tremor of whatever sort, Max was going to be taken from him. He couldn't or indeed wouldn't allow this.

In conclusion, Henry was forcing a re-appraisal of this person who had shared an ambulance from Brittas Bay up to Loughlinstown. In the ambulance, Henry had appeared a general nine to sixer, a person of no real consequence and, if truth be known, an individual who had no obvious outstanding reason to be considered as anyone special. But now, this same individual had commandeered a television show with the significance of The Late-Late and now was coming into actuality the need for a re-appraisal.

His father had assured him that a separation would not have taken effect, but he had tempered this by declaring that he had wished Peter to have been more available with pertinent information concerning goings on in Brittas Bay. Had he been alluding to the rescuing of Henry, or Max having a heart upset of whatever magnitude? Almost at once Peter was going to have to provide himself with a satisfactory answer.

Peter, whilst having insinuated that Henry may very well wish to partake in a game of his primary love – football, was searching his parents' faces for signs of either their approval or disapproval. He was unable to settle on either and elected to follow Henry and his lead in whatever was going to happen next.

Henry, available for every viewer, had proposed a uniting of their two personae, in order to promote (or substantiate) the concern of M.S. throughout an arc of alluded world appreciation and this was causing him a degree of bother. If he was to accept and move ahead with this suggestion then his individual isolation would in effect come to an end. But was his condition of more importance than a revelation to the world of the interest being shown for this same concern? He had to face a situation of conjecture and having to guess about things which had never affected him before.

Max, of course, was a consideration to be brought to the fore. He was immediately a guide dog. What he had done was to rescue an individual who had been drowning. It was literally a case of nothing more and nothing less. But with this new circumstance coming to the fore, things could be seen to be about to change. He had the propensity to become an icon in the (hoped for) subjection and possible eradication of Multiple-Sclerosis and if this was going to occur, Peter was going to have to put aside any intended involvement with Max on a one to one existence. But was he bigger than his immediate intended involvement with the endearing golden Labrador? Questions, questions, questions.

Peter, being the responsible human whom his parents had instigated with a bigger understanding of concerns other than merely himself, rose to the fore. He enquired of Henry his intentions for the foreseeable future, given Peter and his agreeing forbearance to particular proposals. Henry revealed to Peter, his involvement with the world as his playground. Suspecting that Peter (for whatever reason) may actually be unaware of Henry and his significance to the world, went on to reveal to all that he had interests encompassing the entire globe and suggesting that if NASA had furthered their intrusions into space, he may very well have been up there too.

The mention of N.A.S.A. brought an immediate support (of sorts) from Peters' father and he suddenly became an avid silent participant to the evolving proceedings. He had known and recognised who Henry had been, from the outset of the broadcast, but had not appreciated that the rescued individual in Brittas Bay had been someone of the propensity of Henry, his source of info being Dave, who had not met Henry.

"Having the world as a template with which to move around with a certain degree of freedom, I suspect that somewhere within this arena, may be a location with answers to your particular affliction, which may not have been considered heretofore or even within the knowledge of your registered aims". Henry spoke in an unassuming manner and one which was not intended to exert any pressure upon an otherwise non-committed listener such as Peters' father. Helen, understanding her need for non-involvement in any conversation bordering on the alleviating of the situation having a solution to the global awareness of the M.S. criteria, said nothing.

Minutes remained for the ascribed time of the show and Henry was looking for a response from Peter which would allow all those with a shared regard for this affliction, to concede that an approved outcome was going to be forthcoming. Still Peter was stuck in the realms of preponderance. He knew, within himself, what response he would accede to but always there was that self-centeredness that had been a friend to him for the months past; months when the only ally whom he could trust with his initiatives had been his own mentality. Was he really going to break with all of that which he had known to be true, his bond with his dog, to be thrown up and usurped for something as selfish as his own concerns?

Drawing himself up (to the extent that he could) in his wheelchair and with the receiver to his ear, he expostulated by declaring his wish to assist and accompany Henry in whatever endeavours he could bring to bear in the eradication of this sickening and disturbing malady which was, right at that point in time, visiting itself upon the world.

Henry, conceding that without this stance having been taken by Peter, the entire show would have had a certain virtuosity over which he would have had no control.

At this point in time, the show concluded and what was to happen was able to take place. Henry had arranged with Peter to actually meet up and allow progression to evolve. He had enquired as to the meeting taking place and the future availability for Peter to accompany him wherever. Peter had retorted by insinuating that he had been just about to go to The States (in the company of Keith) and that therefore there was no reason for him to be unavailable for whatever. He was quite in agreement (and available) to be away from home for an indeterminate time period. What was he to prepare himself for?

20. Brittas Bay X 2

Henrys' reply had been one of non-committed innuendo. He suggested that Peter would be accompanying him in his proposed itinerary and spreading the message associated with the concerns for M.S., without portraying an immediate cure. He also may have the company of Max.

Time was seen to have elapsed and all things had appeared to fall back into the appreciated position which they could be understood to have occupied in the very beginning. But Henry was left with one confusing issue which had perplexed him from the outset. He was intent on finding out the circumstances which had led to him being in the ambulance, in the first place.

He had spent a degree of time contemplating over this issue and at the end concurred that finding out may bring into existence, a set of occurrences bringing about a bonding between all parties, which being seen under a different arrangement would never be understood to be capable of producing the required bonding.

Henry now had a new set of acquaintances, people who all were involved with his having usurped The Late-Late Show. They consisted of the initially involved participants and a few peripheral individuals. He had spoken to Peter and Helen on the telephone, he knew of Bill and his training of guide dogs; Dave had entered his area of knowledge as being a taxi-driver of some propensity and Keith had some tangible association with the assembled masses. He had come to know of the importance of Peter's father in the situation and there was someone called Tim who would bear recognition. There was a pair of ambulance personnel who had had an imput and he had come to know that the dog had arrived originally from Trish's house.

As he considered all the attendant masses, he sought to bring into existence a situation where they could all come together. Thinking about it for long enough, he finally resolved on a solution. The one individual, who was, certainly expected to be there, was Max. Everything transpiring was going to occur around him. Max had rescued him and Max was going to form a centre for all the others to partake of a re-enactment. He wanted to know of a possible reason for all that had occurred.

He had telephoned down to Peter's house and had spoken with his dad. Simply, he had put it to him that a re-enactment was being planned but could he appreciate a situation where Peter could be kept unaware of the entire picture. Peter was going to be required but in such a way as to allow him to feel that this was going to simply be something between Peter (himself) and Henry – very low key.

Could he arrange for the other Wexford participants to be assembled in Brittas Bay on an appropriate date? Peter's dad assured Henry that this was well within his range of capability. Henry was so fixed in his cunning plan that he resolved for several things to happen, all together, on the respective date. His aim was to surprise a large proportion of the assembled masses.

To do this, he was going to make use of all of the people who had contributed towards having saved his life. Max obviously was the pivot around which everything had occurred and now Henry was going to reveal his unending gratitude for this event. He was going to bring about an event which would allow all participants to appreciate their association and closeness.

Henry with all his kudos had selected to take over the North Car Park area and bring into existence a barbeque for all concerned. Individually he had contacted all relevant parties and having secured support for his proposal, it all looked good. He had also, after consultation with Bill, arranged for a senior veterinary consultant to be in attendance for the benefit of Max. A catering company had been coerced into providing expected arrangements for the event. The only unknown for the entire occasion remained The Weather.

Planning continued and the weather was elected to be left in the hands of whomever. What could be resolved was and Peter had been contacted to re-enact the event purely for the amusement of Henry. He had been unaware of further proceedings and thought that events on the day were simply going to revolve around himself and Henry.

For one day, immediately before the proposed event, Max had been 'borrowed' from Peter. He had been brought to Bill, who had been delighted to be reacquainted with the adorable golden Labrador and a complete make-over had been the resultant outcome. Coat brushed, nails trimmed and mouth prepared for upcoming smiles (photo opportunity). Bill, as a result of his regard for Max, had had him go through a complete medical and Max had come through the same having passed on all accounts – no evidence of any heart condition.

The day arrived and as it had turned out the day in question was revealing itself to be one of glorious sunshine. Henry had managed to cordon off the area of The North Car Park (by requesting a closing of the area for the purpose of filming). It being a public area and always having to be available for public access, particular approval had to be obtained for the entire proposed event to occur. Again with Henry and his perceived personae, this was no problem and so The North Car Park area became just another area for Henry to involve himself with, in order to play.

From early on the required personnel had been arriving at the car park area and directed onto the beach. Far from only involving the people expected these people had brought along numerous other bodies. They had wished everyone and his brother to understand that they had been requested by Henry to be in attendance. "So let's all descend on Brittas Bay, for whatever", had been the feeling.

Henry (or rather his team of officials) was directing people down onto the beach hoping to recreate a full beach of Dublin's overspill – it being a glorious day. Everyone had to be in a position of having their back to the entrance to the beach from the car park and not to reveal any surprise (or expression) upon Peter's arrival.

An area had been set apart for the construction of a giant barbeque area and cooking was commencing. Odours of cooking rose around the area and smells of grilling moved around it; producing a desire for food from all participants. Amidst the conniving appearance it was suddenly being disclosed that Peter was in the immediate vicinity and that things were shortly to come about.

Henry was parading all around and stressing the need for secrecy to be preserved. Dave had brought Peter to Brittas Bay and having been made a part of the conspiracy he was playing it to the extent of merely delivering Peter and Max down to the car park area and then going away in order to conduct other business (and he'd be back later). He had merely left the car park area, doubled back and then headed down in order to be just one more of a faceless crowd sitting in a fixed position on the same beach. An enormous number of hats were being worn and regarding the beach from the car park, few features could be discerned in order to belie the presence of Peter's acquaintances.

The word was out; Peter had arrived. As the pair came onto the beach, the drone of a helicopter split the air and came into view; from the Dublin direction.

It hovered briefly over the water and then, skilfully the pilot brought her down on the beach. The Perspex door flew to one side and Keith stepped out.

As Henry had done an appraisal of all of Peter's contacts and acquaintances, he had discovered that one name represented a friend who had gone across to The States in order to find out the situation pertaining to wheelchair mobility and access. Peter, having gained a scholarship to a university in The States, required this information and Keith had gone across in order to gain the same. Henry had got in touch with him and knowing the magnitude of what he had been proposing to bring into effect, urged Keith to come back, especially for the event. Coming in, he had sized up what was happening on the beach and his appraisal being correct, he knew where to go, after leaving the helicopter; he wound his way over towards Peter.

Peter had recognised that an aircraft was in the immediate area and held back in his descent onto the beach. Keith had hit the beach running. He left the 'copter and ran towards his friend. He had been told all about Peter and his condition (or suspected improvement) from various uninformed sources and, frankly, hadn't known what to believe. He saw a wheelchair being accompanied by a guide dog, a large pile of crumpled blankets on the same, but from a distance he was unable to detect a sign of his friend. As he ran (slower), the blankets moved to reveal the remaining substance of his once athletically endower companion. He was however delighted to see him.

Having got up to him, he held out his hand. When he had last seen Peter, arm movement had been available and in no way was Keith prepared for the sight greeting him. Slumped down inside the wheelchair and completely supported by the confines of the same, Peter was now demonstrating only having the use of his head. His entire body appeared to be the subject of Peter's mental appreciation of being a candidate suffering from M.S. and "things were only going to get worse".

Peter was holding the opinion that he had been visited with this malady and that therefore he should see himself as someone such as, his appreciation of Stephen Hawkins was and therefore he had better only be a voice (or similar). He really had no right to a physical presence of any kind and life ought to be conducted from the security of his own room (aw, poor me).

Having got to him, Keith sized up the situation and conceded that his information pertinent to The USA was now appearing irrelevant and out of date; things were much worse than he had known or even suspected. He looked his friend in the eye and announced his delight at being home. Peter looked at him, out of the tangle of blankets and smiled. Max closed in towards the wheelchair, knowing his responsibility for Peter whilst still knowing that the fresh inclusion to his area of immediate concern now included his previous (and recognised) initial contact with the human race. Max was delighted to be seeing Keith again.

The trio made their way onto the beach and there they were met by the enthusiastic presence of Henry. He had been party to the arrival of the helicopter and had previously planned for the meeting between Peter and Keith (so far no surprises). Peter, regarding and recognising Henry amidst all the beachcombers present, standing with their backs to him, also recognised another figure. Recognising a shirt, which he had seen only minutes before, he struggled to put a face to the available back presenting figure – Dave! This was something which he recognised as being impossible; Dave had left him minutes earlier, bound for other business. "Something smelt in Denmark". He moved the wheelchair in the direction of the figure and Dave aware that this movement had come about; turned.

Immediately upon this recognition being made, everyone turned, "SURPRISE", faces were given to all of the assembled masses and Peter was aware that the entire beach was taken up with people whom he had known directly. They all closed down around him and salutations were exchanged. It was at this stage that Peter suspected that something of which he had been unaware was happening. Henry came over towards him and eagerly welcomed him to the beach.

"Welcome".

He turned and brought Peter over towards the Barbeque. Getting to the aroma emanating location, Peter was demonstrating his enthusiasm by drawing himself up slightly in the wheelchair. Keith was watching all this with interest and had moved down to this area, down on the right hand side in the company of Max. Stroking the dog with enthusiasm and the movement being reciprocated warmly, it could have been that the separation between the two had never occurred, the reunification was complete.

Some participants were standing merely watching and appeared to be showing that in reality their presence was surplus to requirements. Henry had stepped in towards Peter and had drawn a tray across the front of the wheelchair. He turned to the barbeque and taking a cut of the pro-offered steak, placed it on a plate and moved it onto the tray. Keith understanding the situation leant forward and taking a knife and fork, he cut the presented steak in order to make it more amenable for Peter and his capabilities for chewing. He gave the steak, in small pieces, to Peter and subtly slipped an occasional piece to Max, who was willing to accept it simply to show his pleasure at this meeting again with his previous associate.

The purpose of the barbeque seemed to have achieved its aim; it had brought about the integration and association of all parties concerned with Henry and his involvement with the ambulance. Questions were being asked amongst all parties and there were answers being disclosed, answers with a small measure of intelligence.

Time had gone by and people had broken up into little groups, each one satisfied with their own level of intelligence. Peter and Henry had moved over towards where the tide had now gone out. They were in an approximate and similar position to where Peter had been prior to events occurring. Henry had asked Peter the stage at which he had become aware of him swimming past. He was interested because he had simply remembered swimming in a relaxed frame of mind, after the pressures of the financial world of Dublin.

Peter went on to say that the first clear indication which he had to show an imagined cause for concern was sight of a single arm, stationary and pointing towards the sky. He couldn't explain his sudden clarity of vision but what he insisted upon was this sudden appreciation of sight being now available to him. He had seen this arm and he had suspected that to the arm there may very well be attached a body. The arm had sunk beneath the surface and almost immediately resurfaced with a body attached, the body had gulped a quantity of air and then sunk again. Fixing his attention on the position where he had last seen body and arm, Max had turned and dived in the area and returned to the surface with the body in question – Henry. Max had then brought himself and the rescued body to the edge of the beach and at the breaking waves had allowed people to take over. He had then returned to the waves and his splashing about. He went on to say that it was at this point that Max had had his heart tremor or whatever – it had never been diagnosed.

Peter (dismissing the significance of his rescue of Max) said that upon Max having being an unconscious body, lying by the breaking waves, it had necessitated in the ambulance being alerted, William (one of the paramedics) had arrived down by Peter's collapsed body and as a result of investigation had returned with a stretcher and the other paramedic (Declan). Together they had brought Peter up to the ambulance while Max had been carried up by an onlooker. It was at this stage Henry might have been expected to know the rest.

Henry revealed that he had no recollection of all this because the ambulance was actually on the way to the hospital before he had come too. His first understanding had been a lick from a golden Labrador and he being further confused because he had known of no rescue service which employed dogs to bring unconscious bodies back to life, as it were. When he had looked further, a youth had been on a stretcher on the opposite side of the ambulance. This youth had been unknown to him and left him wondering if he had died or not, but it was by seeing the youth attempting to talk that he became convinced that he had gone to hell and he was now unable to hear the spoken voice (he could hear the ambulance engine). Confusion, but it all seemed to settle into some sort of understanding when he had engaged in conversation with William (the paramedic).

He had felt enormous relieve when they had got to the hospital, the engine had stopped and the youth could finally get words together revealing his propensity with M.S.; Henry now had the knowledge which he had been looking for as regards occurrences having happened around the beach. He was seeing the duo with a fresh insight and placing a value upon his own life which was suggesting to all, that he, Henry, did indeed have a value outside of his imagined understanding.

Questions were remaining that simple logic couldn't answer; how had a single youth (and a youth with the debilitation of M.S.) been the only person to appreciate his predicament? What had allowed the youth to simply observe the incident and whilst being unable to physically render aid himself, have a dog with the savvy of Max? All these questions were going to have to remain speculation and allow Henry to appreciate that fate had played a role in all the events which had transpired. This episode had been meant to happen and so now he must play his part in bringing about the next development so that satisfaction may be seen to be the resultant outcome.

Together Henry and Peter were looking out across the sea; each lost amidst their own individual thoughts. Understanding that a significant member of this entire occurrence was the dog (now splashing away with abandon to their front) and obviously searching for another Henry, in order to re-enact the entire event again and have a degree of freedom. As Max frolicked, smashing the waves with his paws, he kept an eye out for his primary concern and when Peter commanded (at Henry's suggestion) that Max come in to heel, this was what had been performed immediately.

At Peter's command Max came immediately in to the heel position, waiting for further commands. They came and Max found himself being accompanied off to face examination from the vet whom Henry had arranged to be in attendance. There was a low table at one side of the barbeque and Max was commanded to get on to the top of it. He did and then being commanded to lie down; did that also. Complete with stethoscope and with an abundance of time, the vet proceeded to give Max an 'all over'. This was something which had already been performed at the training centre under the instruction of Bill.

It must be understood that the results (or answers) to a lot of these proceedings were already within the grasp of the person who had brought this repast into existence   Henry suggested that a form of Presentation was about to commence.   He was bringing into existence a situation where they were all collectively meeting around the barbeque. He called for attention. People straining to catch a glimpse of what he was saying, congregated around the same barbeque.

"I want you all to know that it is with a very great intention that I have gathered you all here today. The purpose for it all is resting here in front of me, on his four legs. It is only by allowing a fuss and indeed commendation to be made of Max that further awareness can constructively be shown that it is indeed relevant in other areas also"

"Ladies and Gentlemen, it is with the greatest of pleasure that I ask you to put your hands together and allow appreciation for all the effort — known and unknown, to be extended towards training facilities which will cater towards producing this very much needed facility, which is proving to be of such a benefit to all incumbents accepting upon themselves a disability of whatever sort. It is my turn now to show my gratitude for this work by presenting in recognition of my appreciation, a monetary Thank-You to a representative who will stand for all involved in the work being done in this direction. I give you Bill and thank you".

This had not been expected and caught the dog handler completely off guard. Stuffing his face with food which had being prepared on the barbeque and expecting Henry's little diatribe to be contending with other issues, Bill had subjected himself to getting as much food into his mouth, in the shortest time possible (knowing that this event was not going to occur again) and therefore when attention had been extended in his direction he was completely unable to say anything. Amidst spluttering and guffawing he came to the fore. Henry had reached under the table beside the barbeque and withdrawn a number of envelopes. Standing tall, he handed one of these towards Bill, who in his genuine embarrassment and amidst his involvement with half-digested food, meekly accepted the same.

Giving himself time to swallow the remaining food in his mouth, he paused; in order to swallow and opened the envelope. Staring at the contained cheque, he first looked at it and then at Henry. "I think you may have made a mistake". "No mistake! It is an expression of my gratitude". Bill in his amazement waved the paper in the air and it was seen to be a cheque for €50,000.

Silence had befallen the assembled people and being unaware of such generosity, especially in the current economic times, a small understanding was being extended towards the appreciation of Henry and his wealth. Gratefully withdrawing from a position of being the centre of attention and firmly clutching the enclosed piece of paper, Bill lost himself amidst the masses allowing Henry to continue.

"The next presentation which I am going to make can be seen to be unusual, unusual but required. It is a mark of my thanks to all those who in any way came together, on the day in question and allowed me the gift of life. It is with the greatest of pleasure that I now make a presentation to the ambulance service and ask William (I think it is) and Declan to step forward".

The two paramedics had not been expecting this and now understanding that they were going to have to represent all ambulance personnel throughout the country, they came to the fore. William extending his hand was given a second envelope which in his appreciation, he opened. It contained a cheque for €100,000.

At this stage awe had seized the spectators and all were left feeling wonderment as to what was going to follow. Henry now took out a pile of loosely assembled papers and turning in order to address the throng stated that another obvious candidate for his disposal of 'trinkets' (which got a laugh) was Max; however, he disclosed, Max did not have the physical propensity to actually receive what Henry was going to give to him. It might be understood that Peter should do the receiving on this occasion. Yeah!

As Henry gathered all the papers into an understood pile, Peter had understood the need for him to possibly stand in order to receive whatever Henry was going to make available for him/Max. He thought about things and realised that as far as he was concerned there was no way in which he was going to control a situation whereby he was going to stand. For months now he had only allowed himself to know that he was only getting worse; there was no tangible reason for the Brittas Bay occurrence, or what had revealed itself at home. He was still stuck within his own mind-set. He could only look as far as himself and by doing so – no answer!

Then it occurred to him; he was seeing. His eyesight had been renewing itself and now was at such a level, if not as it had originally been, it was a great deal better than he had recently been experiencing. Now he was asking himself for the truth of which Keith had talked of months before. Was his having this upsetting disability all for a purpose? Could he accept that having this condition and having been personally aware of it, he could now become a champion for all incumbents similarly afflicted? Had his life achieved a purpose? As a result of his own self-centeredness, of the last few months, he had been unable to see a bigger effect.

He shut all thoughts out of his mind and realising that the event of that time was for the benefit of his one true companion, his friend and so; let's celebrate. Henry finished gathering the papers together and straightening himself, faced Peter.

"The first thing which I wish to reveal to you is that Max has now received a certificate allowing the world to know that he no longer has a heart condition. He has attained a clean bill of health and in answer to what you may be about to ask, How? It seems that the massage which he was given immediately following his collapse, moved the obstruction from his arterial passage and it is now of no concern whatever. He can, in all confidence, assume life as a guide dog with no disability whatsoever". It was at this juncture that Bill stepped forward, "And may I add that with all confidence, we are more than willing to accept Max back into the centre in order for him to pass out as fully certified and in possession of an appropriate C.V. to accompany him wherever".

All around, cheers were shouted and cries of congratulations were extended towards the dog now contentedly resting against the right front wheel of Peter's chair. Peter smiled and thought with satisfaction that the dog –his dog, appeared to have now moved from death to life. Gone was the proverbial shadow which had always accompanied Max everywhere; he hadn't completed his guide dog training, he'd failed his medical, he was going to die – sooner rather than later. But now, a complete translation, a reprieve, a new chance at life and all because of a massage which had given him a fresh hold on something that was going to allow him that extra time frame to fulfil his life's purpose. Max was one of a kind, a friend who made no demands, who had been brought back from the very proximity of death by as simple a thing as a massage.

Henry continued; "You can see that I have here in my hands a lot more than a simple bill of health and it is with significant praise and thanks, towards a certain dog, that I now extend my second piece of literature. It is a dogs passport, a passport which will allow Max to accompany whoever, wherever and this I can only look forward too. A guide dog with all the virtues which Max displays is something which can only be seen to be a bonus. He is loved by all. So thank you, Max".

Henry waved the certificate in the air and continued, "He has to go somewhere and have someone to go with him, Ladies and Gentlemen, and I now allow you to know that in a very short space of time, a team whom I will refer to as 'The New Fab Four' will be heading for pastures new. Peter, Keith, Max and I are going abroad and showing the concern that Ireland has for a condition such as M.S... We may never move, revealing a cure for this condition, but we will move forward showing to all that a country with the identity of Ireland can champion the cause and investigate the concerns which this condition entails. This final piece of paper which I am now holding is a piece of paper confirming flight times and procedures for The New Fab Four. I now give them to Peter".

He was leaning over in the direction of the wheelchair when Peter fixed him with a grin and clutching the arms of the chair, rose up. He shuffled towards him and with no thought for what he was doing, grasped the papers being held towards him.

Behind him two men (one being Tim and the other Peter's father) stood transfixed by the occurring event and one leaning in towards the other said "And soon there may not be a need for any wheelchairs, eh Graham"?